AF514739

Tucholsky Wagner Zola Scott Sydow Schlegel
Turgenev Wallace Fonatne Freud
Twain Walther von der Vogelweide Fouqué Friedrich II. von Preußen
Weber Freiligrath Frey
Fechner Fichte Weiße Rose von Fallersleben Kant Ernst Richthofen Frommel
Hölderlin
Engels Fielding
Fehrs Faber Flaubert Eichendorff Tacitus Dumas
Maximilian I. von Habsburg Fock Eliasberg Zweig Ebner Eschenbach
Feuerbach Ewald Eliot Vergil
Goethe London
Mendelssohn Balzac Shakespeare Elisabeth von Österreich Ganghofer
Lichtenberg Rathenau Dostojewski
Trackl Stevenson Tolstoi Hambruch Doyle Gjellerup
Mommsen Thoma Lenz Hanrieder Droste-Hülshoff
Dach Verne von Arnim Hägele Hauff Humboldt
Reuter
Karrillon Garschin Rousseau Hagen Hauptmann Gautier
Damaschke Defoe Hebbel Baudelaire
Descartes
Wolfram von Eschenbach Dickens Schopenhauer Hegel Kussmaul Herder
Bronner Darwin Melville Grimm Jerome Rilke George
Campe Horváth Aristoteles Bebel Proust
Bismarck Vigny Gengenbach Barlach Voltaire Federer Herodot
Heine
Storm Casanova Lessing Tersteegen Gilm Grillparzer Georgy
Chamberlain Langbein Gryphius
Brentano Lafontaine
Strachwitz Claudius Schiller Kralik Iffland Sokrates
Katharina II. von Rußland Bellamy Schilling
Gerstäcker Raabe Gibbon Tschechow
Löns Hesse Hoffmann Gogol Wilde Gleim Vulpius
Luther Heym Hofmannsthal Klee Hölty Morgenstern Goedicke
Roth Heyse Klopstock Kleist
Luxemburg Puschkin Homer Mörike
La Roche Horaz Musil
Machiavelli
Navarra Aurel Musset Kierkegaard Kraft Kraus
Lamprecht Kind Kirchhoff Hugo Moltke
Nestroy Marie de France
Nietzsche Nansen Laotse Ipsen Liebknecht
Marx Ringelnatz
von Ossietzky Lassalle Gorki Klett Leibniz
May vom Stein Lawrence Irving
Petalozzi Platon Knigge
Sachs Poe Pückler Michelangelo Kock Kafka
Liebermann Korolenko
de Sade Praetorius Mistral Zetkin

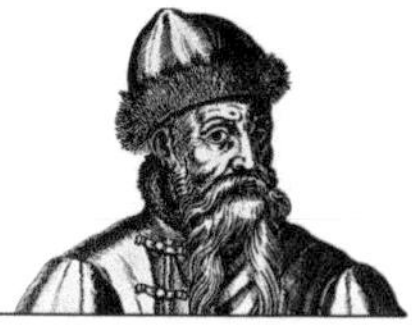

Disturbances of the Heart

Oliver T. (Oliver Thomas) Osborne

Imprint

This book is part of the TREDITION CLASSICS series.

Author: Oliver T. (Oliver Thomas) Osborne
Cover design: toepferschumann, Berlin (Germany)

Publisher: tredition GmbH, Hamburg (Germany)
ISBN: 978-3-8491-9119-1

www.tredition.com
www.tredition.de

DISTURBANCES OF THE HEART

Discussion of the Treatment of the Heart in Its Various Disorders, With a Chapter on Blood Pressure

OLIVER T. OSBORNE, A.M., M.D.
Professor of Therapeutics and formerly Professor of Clinical Medicine in Yale Medical School NEW HAVEN, CONN.

THE JOURNAL of AMERICAN MEDICAL ASSOCIATION
Five Hundred Thirty-Five
North Dearborn Street, Chicago

PREFACE

The second edition of this book is offered with the hope that it will be as favorably received as was the former edition, The text has been carefully revised, in a few parts deleted, and extensively elaborated to bring the book up to the present knowledge concerning the scientific therapy of heart disturbances. A complete section has been added on blood pressure.

PREFACE TO THE FIRST EDITION

That marvelous organ which, moment by moment and year by year, keeps consistently sending the blood on its path through the arteriovenous system is naturally one whose structure and function need to be carefully studied if one is to guard it when threatened by disease. This series of articles deals with heart therapy, not discussing the heart structurally and anatomically, but taking up in detail the various forms of the disturbances which may affect the heart. The cordial reception given by the readers of The Journal to this series of articles has warranted its issue in book form so that it may be slipped into the pocket for review at appropriate times, or kept on the desk for convenient reference.

CONTENTS

DISTURBANCES OF THE HEART IN GENERAL

Of prime importance in the treatment of diseases of the heart is a determination of the exact, or at least approximately exact, condition of its structures and a determination of its ability to work.

This is not the place to describe its anatomy or its nervous mechanism or the newer instruments of precision in estimating the heart function, but they may be briefly itemized. It has now been known for some time that the primary stimulus of cardiac contraction generally occurs at the upper part of the right auricle, near its junction with the superior vena cava, and that this region may be the "timer" of the heart.

This is called the sinus node, or the sino-auricular node, and consists of a small bundle of fibers resembling muscle tissue. Lewis [Footnote: Lewis: Lecture in the Harvey Society, New York Academy of Medicine, Oct. 31, 1914.] describes this bundle as from 2 to 3 cm. in length, its upper end being continuous with the muscle fibers of the wall of the superior vena cava. Its lower end is continuous with the muscle fibers of the right auricle. From this node "the excitation wave is conducted radially along the muscular strands at a uniform rate of about a thousand millimeters per second to all portions of the auricular musculature."

Though a wonderfully tireless mechanism, this region may fall out of adjustment, and the stimuli proceeding from it may not be normal or act normally. It has been shown recently not only that there must be perfection of muscle, nerve and heart circulation but also that the various elements in solution in the blood must be in perfect amounts and relationship to each other for the heart stimulation to be normal. It has also been shown that if for any reason this region of the right auricle is disturbed, a stimulus or impulse might come from some other part of the auricle, or even from the ventricle, or from some point between them. Such stimulations may constitute auricular, ventricular or auriculoventricular extra contractions or extrasystoles, as they are termed. In the last few years it has been discovered that the auriculoventricular handle, or "bundle of His," has a necessary function of conductivity of auricular impulse to ventricular contraction. A temporary disturbance of this conductivity will cause a heart block, an intermittent disturbance will cause intermittent heart block (Stokes-Adams disease), and a prolonged disturbance, death. It has also been shown that extrasystoles, meaning irregular heart action, may be caused by impulses originating at the apex, at the base or at some point in the right ventricle.

In the ventricles, Lewis states, the Purkinje fibers act as the conducting agent, stimuli being conducted to all portions of the endocardium simultaneously at a rate of from 2,000 to 1,000 mm. per second. The ventricular muscle also aids in the conduction of the stimuli, but at a slower rate, 300 mm. per minute. The rate of conduction, Lewis believes, depends on the glycogen content of the structures, the Purkinje fibers, where conduction is most rapid, containing the largest amount of glycogen, the auricular musculature containing the next largest amount of glycogen, and the ventricular muscle fibers the least amount of glycogen.

Anatomists and histologists have more perfectly demonstrated the muscle fibers of the heart and the structure at and around the valves; the physiologic chemists have shown more clearly the action of drugs, metals and organic solutions on the heart; and the physiologists and clinicians with laboratory facilities have demonstrated by various new apparatus the action of the heart and the circulatory power under various conditions. It is not now sufficient to state that the heart is acting irregularly, or that the pulse is irregular; the endeavor should be to determine whit causes the irregularity, and what kind of irregularity is present.

CLINICAL INTERPRETATION OF PULSE TRACINGS

A moment may be spent on clinical interpretation of pulse tracings. It has recently been shown that the permanently irregular pulse is due to fibrillary contraction, or really auricular fibrillation—in other words, irregular stimuli proceeding from the auricle—and that such an irregular pulse is not due to disturbance at the auriculoventricular node, as believed a short time ago. These little irregular stimuli proceeding from the auricle reach the auriculoventricular node and are transmitted to the ventricle as rapidly as the ventricle is able to react. Such rapid stimuli may soon cause death; or, if for any reason, medicinal or otherwise, the ventricle becomes indifferent to these stimuli, it may not take note of more than a certain portion of the stimuli. It then acts slowly enough to allow prolongation of life, and even considerable activity. If such a heart becomes more rapid from such stimuli, 110 or more, for any length of time, the condition becomes very serious. Digitalis in such a condition is, of course, of supreme value on account of its ability to slow the heart. Such irregularity perhaps most frequently occurs with valvular disease, especially mitral stenosis and in the muscular degenerations of senility, as fibrosis.

Atropin has been used to differentiate functional heart block from that produced by a lesion. Hart [Footnote: Hart: Am. Jour. Med. Sc., 1915, cxlix, 62.] has used atropin in three different types of heart block. In the first the heart block is induced by digitalis. This was entirely removed by atropin. In the second type, where there was normal auricular activity, but where the ventricular contractions were decreased, atropin affected an increase in the number of ventricular contractions, but did not completely remove the heart block. He adopted atropin where the heart block was associated with auricular fibrillation. The number of ventricular contractions was increased, but not enough to indicate the complete removal of the heart block.

Lewis [Footnote: Lewis: Brit. Med. Jour., 1909, ii, 1528.] believes that 50 percent of cardiac arrhythmia originates in muscle disturbance or incoordination in the auricle. These stimuli are irregular in intensity, and the contractions caused are irregular in degree. If the wave lengths of the pulse tracing show no regularity- -if, in fact, hardly two adjacent wave lengths are alike—the disturbance is auricular fibrillation. Injury to the auricle, or pressure for any reason on the auricle, may so disturb the transmission of stimuli and contractions that the contractions of the ventricle are very much fewer than the stimuli proceeding from the auricle. In other words, a form of heart block may occur. Various stimuli coming through the pneumogastric nerves, either from above or from the peripheral endings in the stomach or intestines, may inhibit or slow the ventricular contractions. It seems to have been again shown, as was earlier understood, that there are inhibitory and accelerator ganglia in the heart itself, each subject to various kinds of stimulation and various kinds of depression.

Both auricular fibrillation and auricular flutter are best shown by the polygraph and the electrocardiograph. The former is more exact as to details. Auricular flutter, which has also been called auricular tachysystole, is more common that is supposed. It consists of rapid coordinate auricular contractions, varying from 200 to 300 per minute. Fulton [Footnote: Fulton, F. T.: "Auricular Flutter," with a Report of Two Cases, Arch. Int. Med., October, 1913, p. 475.] finds in this condition that the initial stimulus arises in some part of the auricular musculature other than the sinus node. It is different from paroxysmal tachycardia, in which the heart rate rarely exceeds 180 per minute. In auricular flutter there is always present a certain amount of heart block, not all the stimuli reaching the ventricle. There may be a ratio of auricular contractions to ventricular contractions, according to Fulton, of 2:1, 3:1, 4:1 and 5:1, the 2:1 ratio being most common.

Of course it is generally understood that children have a higher pulse rate than adults; that women normally have a higher pulse rate than men at the same age; that strenuous muscular exercise, frequently repeated, without cardiac tire while causing the pulse to be rapid at the time, slows the pulse during the interim of such exercise and may gradually cause a more or less permanent slow pulse. It should be remembered that athletes have slow pulse, and the severity of their condition must not be interpreted by the rate of the pulse. Even with high fever the pulse of an athlete may be slow.

Not enough investigations have been made of the rate of the pulse during sleep under various conditions. Klewitz [Footnote: Klewitz: Deutsch. Arch. f. klin. Med. 1913, cxii, 38.] found that the average pulse rate of normal individuals while awake and active was 74 per minute, but while asleep the average fell to 59 per minute. He found also that if a state of perfect rest could be obtained during the waking period, the pulse rate was slowed. This is also true in cases of compensated cardiac lesions, but it was not true in decompensated hearts. He found that irregularities such as extrasystoles and organic tachycardia did not disappear during sleep, whereas functional tachycardia did.

It is well known that high blood pressure slows the pulse rate; that low blood pressure generally increases the pulse rate, and that arteriosclerosis, or the gradual aging of the arteries, slows the pulse, except when the cardiac degeneration of old age makes the heart again more irritable and more rapid. The rapid heart in hyperthyroidism is also well understood. It is not so frequently noted that hypersecretion of the thyroid may cause a rapid heart without any other tangible or discoverable thyroid symptom or symptoms of hyperthyroidism. Bile in the blood almost always slows the pulse.

INTERPRETATION OF TRACINGS

The interpretation of the arterial tracing shows that the nearly vertical tip-stroke is due to the sudden rise of blood pressure caused by the contraction of the ventricles. The long and irregular downstroke means a gradual fall of the blood pressure. The first upward rise in this gradual decline is due to the secondary contraction and expansion of the artery; in other words, a tidal wave. The second upward rise in the decline is called the recoil, or the dicrotic wave, and is due to the sudden closure of the aortic valves and the recoil of the blood wave. The interpretation of the jugular tracing, or phlebogram as the vein tracing may be termed, shows the apex of the rise to be due to the contraction of the auricle. The short downward curve from the apex means relaxation of the auricle. The second lesser rise, called the carotid wave, is believed to be due to the impact of the sudden expansion of the carotid artery. The drop of the wave tracing after this cartoid rise is due to the auricular diastole. The immediate following second rise not so high as that of the auricular contraction is known as the ventricular wave, and corresponds to the dicrotic wave in the radial. The next lesser decline shows ventricular diastole, or the heart rest. A tracing of the jugular vein shows the activity of the right side of the heart. The tracing of the carotid and radial shows the activity of the left side of the heart. After normal tracings have been carefully taken and studied by the clinician or a laboratory assistant, abnormalities in these readings are readily shown graphically. Especially characteristic are tracings of auricular fibrillation and those of heart block.

TESTS OF HEART STRENGTH

If both systolic and diastolic blood pressure are taken, and the heart strength is more or less accurately determined, mistakes in the administration of cardiac drugs will be less frequent. Besides mapping out the size of the heart by roentgenoscopy and studying the contractions of the heart with the fluoroscope, and a detailed study of sphygmographic and cardiographic tracings, which methods are not available to the large majority of physicians, there are various methods of approximately, at least, determining the strength of the heart muscle.

Barringer [Footnote: Barringer, T. B., Jr.: The Circulatory Reaction to Graduated Work as a Test of the Heart's Functional Capacity, Arch. Int. Med., March, 1916, p. 363.] has experimented both with normal persons and with patients who were suffering some cardiac insufficiency. He used both the bicycle ergometer and dumb-bells, and finds that there is a rise of systolic pressure after ordinary work, but a delayed rise after very heavy work, in normal persons. In patients with cardiac insufficiency he finds there is a delayed rise in the systolic pressure after even slight exercise, and those with marked cardiac insufficiency have even a lowering of blood pressure from the ordinary level. They all have increase in pulse rate. He quotes several authorities as showing that during muscle work the carbon dioxid of the blood is increased in amount, which, stimulating the nervous centers controlling the suprarenal glands, increases the epinephrin content of the blood. The consequence is contraction of the splanchnic blood vessels, with a rise in general blood pressure. Also, the quickened action of the heart increases the blood pressure. After a rest from the exercise, the extra amount of carbon dioxid is eliminated from the blood, the suprarenal glands decrease their activity, and the blood pressure falls.

Nicolai and Zuntz [Footnote: Nicolai anal Zuntz: Berl. klin. Wehnschr., May 4, 1914, p. 821.] have shown that with the first strain of heavy work the heart increases in size, but it soon becomes normal, or even smaller, as it more strenuously contracts, and the cavities of the heart will be completely emptied at each systole. If the work is too heavy, and the systolic blood pressure is rapidly increased, it may become so great as to prevent the left ventricle from completely evacuating its content. The heart then increases in size and may sooner or later become strained; if this strain is severe, an acute dilatation may of course occur, even in an otherwise well person. Such instances are not infrequent. A heart which is already enlarged or slightly dilated and insufficient, under the stress of muscular labor will more slowly increase its forcefulness, and we have the delayed rise in systolic pressure.

Barringer concludes that:

The pulse rate and the blood pressure reaction to graduated work is a valid test of the heart's functional capacity. If the systolic pressure reaches its greatest height not immediately after work, but from thirty to 120 seconds later, or if the pressure immediately after work is lower than the original level, that work, whatever its amount, has overtaxed the heart's functional capacity and may be taken as an accurate measure of the heart's sufficiency.

In another article, Barringer [Footnote: Barringer, T. B., Jr.: Studies of the Heart's Functional Capacity as Estimated by the Circulatory Reaction to Graduated Work, Arch. Int. Med., May, 1916, p. 670.] advises the use of a 5-pound dumb-bell extended upward from the shoulder for 2 feet. Each such extension represents 10 foot- pounds of work, although the exertion of holding the dumb-bell during the nonextension period is not estimated. He believes that if circulatory tire is shown with less than 100 foot-pounds per minute exercise, other signs of cardiac insufficiency will be in evidence. He also believes that these foot-pound tests can be made to determine whether a patient should be up and about, and also that such graded exercise will increase the heart strength in cardiac insufficiency.

Schoonmaker, [Footnote: Schoonmaker: Am. Jour. Med. Sc., October, 1915, p. 582.] after studying the blood pressure of 127 patients, concludes that myocardial efficiency will be shown by a comparison of the systolic and diastolic blood pressure, with the patient lying down and standing up, after walking a short distance. Such slight exercise should not cause any subjective symptoms, either dyspnea, palpitation or chest pain. If the heart muscle is in good condition, the systolic pressure should remain the same after this slight exertion and these changes in posture. When the heart is good, there may be slight increased pressure when the patient is standing. If, after this slight exercise in the erect posture, the systolic pressure is diminished, the heart muscle is defective.

Martinet [Footnote: Martinet: Presse med., Jan. 20, 1916.] tests the heart strength as follows: He counts the pulse until for two successive minutes there is the same number of beats, first when the patient is lying down, and then when he is standing. He also takes the systolic and diastolic pressures at the same time. He then causes the person to bend rapidly at the knees twenty times. The pulse rate and the blood pressure are then taken each minute for from three to five minutes. The person then reclines, and the pulse and pressure are again recorded, Martinet says that an examination of these records in the form of a chart gives a graphic demonstration of the heart strength. If the heart is weak, there are likely to be asystoles, and tachycardia may occur, or a lowered blood pressure.

Rehfisch [Footnote: Rehfisch: Berl. klin. Wehnsehr., Nov. 29, 1915] states that when a healthy person takes even slight exercise, the aortic closure becomes louder than the second pulmonic sound, showing an increased systolic pressure. If the left ventricle is unable properly to empty itself against the increased resistance ahead, the left auricle will contain too much blood, and with the right ventricle sufficient, there will be an accentuation of the second pulmonic sound and it may become louder than the second aortic sound, showing a cardiac deficiency. If, on the other hand, the right ventricle becomes insufficient, or is insufficient, the second pulmonic sound is weaker than normal, and the prognosis is bad.

Barach [Footnote: Barach: Am. Jour. Med. Sc., July, 1916, p. 84] presents what he terms "the energy index of the circulatory system." He has examined 742 normal persons, and found that the pressure pulse was anywhere from 20 to 80 percent of the diastolic pressure in 80 per cent of his cases, while the average of his figures gave a ratio of 50 percent; but he does not believe that it holds true that in a normal person the pressure pulse equals 50 percent of the diastolic pressure. Barach does not believe we have, as yet, any very accurate method of determining the cardiac strength or circulatory capacity for work. He does not believe that the estimate of the pressure pulse is indicative of cardiac strength. He believes that the important factors in the estimation of the circulatory strength are the systolic pressure, which shows the power of the left ventricle, the diastolic pressure, which shows the intravascular tension during diastole as well as the peripheral resistance, and the pulse rate, which designates the number of times the heart must contract during a minute to maintain the proper flow of blood. He thinks that these three factors are constantly adapting themselves to each other for the needs of the individual, and he finds, for instance, that when the left ventricle is hypertrophied and the output of blood is therefore greater, then the pulse will be slowed. His method of estimation is as follows: For instance, with a systolic pressure of 120 mm. and a diastolic pressure of 80 mm., each pulse beat will represent an energy equal to lifting 120 mm. plus 80 mm., which equals 200 mm. of mercury, and with seventy-two pulse beats the force would be 72 X 200, which equals 14,400 mm. of mercury. He finds an average circulatory strength based on examining 250 normal individuals by the index, which he terms S, D, R (systolic, diastolic rate), to be 20,000 mm. of mercury per minute.

Katzenstein [Footnote: Katzenstein: Deutsch. med. Wehnsehr., April 15, 1915.] finds, after ten years of experience, that the following test of the heart strength is valuable: He records the blood pressure and pulse, and then compresses the femoral artery at Poupart's ligament on the two sides at once. He keeps this pressure up for from two to two and one-half minutes, and then again takes the blood pressure. With a sound heart the blood pressure will be higher and the pulse slower than the previous record taken. If the blood pressure and pulse beat are not changed, it shows that the heart is not quite normal, but not actually incompetent. When the blood pressure is lower and the pulse accelerated, he believes that there is distinct functional disturbance of the heart and loss of power, relatively to the change in pressure and the increase of the pulse rate. He further believes that a heart showing this kind of weakness should, if possible, not be subjected to general anesthesia.

Stange [Footnote: Stange: Russk. Vrach, 1914, xiii. 72.] finds that the cardiac power may be determined by a respiratory test as follows: The patient should sit comfortably, and take a deep inspiration; then he should be told to hold his breath, and the physician compresses the patient's nostrils. As soon as the patient indicates that he can hold his breath no longer, the number of seconds is noted. A normal person should hold his breath from thirty to forty seconds without much subsequent dyspnea, while a patient with myocardial weakness can hold his breath only from ten to twenty seconds, and then much temporary dyspnea will follow. Stange does not find that pulmonary conditions, as tuberculosis, pleurisy or bronchitis, interfere with this test.

Williamson [Footnote: Williamson: Ant. Jour. Med. Sc., April, 1915, p. 492.] believes that we cannot determine the heart strength accurately unless we have some method to note the exact position of the diaphragm, and he has devised a method which he calls the teleroentgen method. With this apparatus he finds that a normal heart responds to exercise within its power by a diminution in size. The same is true of a good compensating pathologic heart. He thinks that a heart which does not so respond by reducing its size after exercise has a damaged muscle, and compensation is more or less impaired.

Practical conclusions to draw from the foregoing suggestions are:

1. An enlargement of the heart after exercise can be well shown only by fluoroscopic examination, and then best by some accurate method of measurement.

2. The blood pressure should be immediately increased by exercise, and after such exercise should soon return to the normal before the exercise. If it goes below the normal the heart is weak, or the exercise was excessive.

3. The pulse rate should increase with exercise, but not excessively, and should within a reasonable time return to normal.

4. The stethoscope will show whether or not the normal sounds of the heart become relatively abnormal after exercise. If such was the fact, though the abnormality was not permanent, heart insufficiency is more or less in evidence.

5. The relation of pulse rate to blood pressure should always be noted, and the working power of the heart may be estimated according to Barach's suggestion.

6. The dumb-bell exercise tests suggested by Barringer (only, the dumb-bells may be of lighter weight) are valuable to note the gradual improvement in heart strength of patients under treatment.

7. The holding the breath test is very suggestive of heart efficiency or weakness, but a series of tests must be made before its limitations are proved.

THE EFFECT OF ATHLETICS ON THE HEART

We can no longer neglect the seriousness of the effects of competitive athletics on the heart, especially in youth and young adults. Not only universities and preparatory schools, but also high schools and even grammar schools must consider the advisability of continuing competitive sports without more control than is now the case. In the first place, the individual is likely to be trained in one particular branch or in one particular line, which develops one particular set of muscles. In the second place, competition to exhaustion, to vomiting, faintness, and even syncope is absolutely inexcusable. Furthermore, contests which partake of brutality should certainly be seriously censored.

A committee appointed some time ago by the Medical Society of the State of California [Footnote: California State Med. Jour., June, 1916 p. 220.] has recently reported its endorsement of Foster's "Indictment of Intercollegiate Athletics." After five years of personal observation of no less than 100 universities and colleges, in thirty-eight states, Foster concludes that intercollegiate athletics have proved a failure, and that they are costly and injurious on account of an excessive physical training of a few students, and of such students as need training least, while healthful and moderate exercise at a small expense for all students is most needed.

Experts, [Footnote: Rubner and Kraus: Vrtljsehr. f. gerichtl. Med, 1914, xlviii, 304.] appointed by the Prussian government to investigate athletics, reported that for physical exercise to be of real value it must be quite different from the preparation of a specially equipped individual trained for a game. Exercise should benefit all children and youth, while athletic prowess necessitates taxing the organism to the limit of endurance, and hence is dangerous and should not be allowed in schools or universities.

McKenzie [Footnote: McKenzie: Am. Jour. Med. Sc., January, 1913, p. 69.] found that exhausting tests of endurance were not adapted to the development of children and youth, because the high blood pressure caused by such exertion soon continued, and he found athletes to have a prolonged increased blood pressure. As is recognized by all, boat racing is particularly bad, especially the 4-mile row. Such severe exertion of course increases the blood pressure, even in these athletes, and the heart increases its speed. There is then exhilaration, later discomfort, and soon, as McKenzie points out, a sensation of constriction in the chest and head. This is soon followed by breathlessness, and soon by a feeling of fulness in the head, and then syncope. The heart, of course, becomes dilated. Heart murmurs are often found after much less severe exertion than boat racing. They may not last long, or they may disappear under proper treatment. He reported that after exercise there were heart murmurs in seventy-four of 266 young men who were in normal health, and that nearly 28 per cent of all normal young men will show a murmur after exercise. He thinks that it is rare to find, after a week, a heart murmur in a previously healthy heart, if the athlete has not passed the age of 30.

There can be no doubt that even one, to say nothing of more, such heart strains is inexcusable and may leave a more or less lasting injury. Such heart strains and exertions are not entirely seen in athletes. A man otherwise well may cause such a heart strain by cranking his automobile, by pumping up a tire, by strenuous lifting, by carrying a load too far or too rapidly, or by running, and an elderly man may even cause such a heart strain by walking, hill climbing, or even golfing, if he does these things. More or less acute dilatation occurring in such persons is likely to recur on the least exertion, unless the patient takes a prolonged rest cure and the heart is so well that it recuperates perfectly. Any chronic myocarditis, however, may prevent such a heart from ever being as perfect as it was before.

Torgersen, [Footnote: Torgersen: Norsk Mag. f. Laegevidensk., April, 1914.] after making 600 examinations of 200 athletes, and 1,200 examinations of members of the rowing crew, decides that it is absolutely essential that there should be skilled daily examinations of every man during training, and a record kept of the condition of his heart, urine, and blood pressure, before and after exercise. When he found albumin in the urine it was always accompanied by a falling of the blood pressure and a rapid heart, with loss of weight and a general feeling of debility.

Middleton [Footnote: Middleton: Am. Jour. Med. Sc., September, 1915, p. 426.] examined students who were training for football, both during the training and after the training period, and found that after the rest succeeding a training period there was an increased systolic and diastolic blood pressure over the records of before the training period. This would tend to indicate some hypertrophy of the heart.

Insurance statistics seem to show that athletes are likely to have earlier cardiovascular-renal disease than other individuals of the same class and occupations.

SUGGESTIONS FOR THE CONTROL OF ATHLETICS

1. Gymnasiums and athletic grounds in connection with all colleges, preparatory schools, seminaries and high schools are essential, and they should be added to grammar schools whenever possible.

2. Physical training and athletic games, and perhaps some type of military training are valuable for the proper development of youth.

3. Some forms of competitive games and some competitive feats are valuable in stimulating training and healthful sports.

4. All competitive sports and all hard training should be under the advice and supervision of a medical council or a medical trainer. Competitive sports which are generally recognized as harmful, mostly on account of their duration as related to the age of the competitors, should be prohibited.

5. Each boy should be carefully examined by a competent physician to decide as to his general health, his limitations and the special training necessary to perfect him or to overcome any defect. Such examinations are even more essential in schools for girls.

6. In all group training, the weak individuals should be noted by the medical trainer, and they should receive special and more carefully graded exercise.

7. In all strenuous training or competitive athletic work, the participators should all be examined more or less frequently and more or less carefully for heart strain and albuminuria and also for a too great increase of blood pressure.

8. All training and all athletic sports should be graded to the age of the boy or girl and not necessarily to his or her size. Many an overgrown boy is injured by athletic prowess beyond his heart strength.

SIGNS OF HEART WEAKNESS

It should be remembered that a normal heart may slow to about 60 during sleep, and all nervous acceleration of the pulse may be differentiated during sleep by the fact that if the heart does not markedly slow, there is cardiac weakness or some general disturbance. There is also cardiac weakness if there is a tendency to yawn or to take long breaths after slight exertions or during exertion, or if there is a feeling of suffocation and the person suddenly wants the windows open, or cannot work, even for a few minutes, in a closed room. If these disturbances are purely functional, exercise not only may be endured, but will relieve some nervous heart disturbances, while it will aggravate a real heart disability. If the heart tends to increase in rapidity on lying down, or the person cannot breathe well or feels suffocated with one ordinary pillow, the heart shows more or less weakness. Extrasystoles are due to abnormal irritability of the heart muscle, and may or may not be noted by the patient. If they are noted, and he complains of the condition, the prognosis is better than though he does not note them.

It has long been known that asthma, emphysema, whooping cough, and prolonged bronchitis with hard coughing will dilate the heart. It has not been recognized until recently, as shown by Guthrie, [Footnote: Guthrie, J. B.: Cough Dilatation Time a Measure of Heart Function, The Journal. A. M. A., Jan. 3, 1914, p. 30.] that even one attack of more or less hard coughing will temporarily enlarge the heart. From these slight occurrences, however, the heart quickly returns to its normal size; but if the coughing is frequently repeated, the dilatation is more prolonged. This emphasizes the necessity of supporting the heart in serious pulmonary conditions, and also the necessity of modifying the intensity of the cough by necessary drugs.

In deciding that a heart is enlarged by noting the apex beat, percussion dulness, and by fluoroscopy, it should be remembered that the apex beat may be several centimeters to the left from the actual normal point, and yet the heart not be enlarged.

The necessity of protecting the heart in acute infections, and the seriousness to the heart of infections are emphasized by the present knowledge that tonsillitis, acute or chronic, and mouth and nose infections of all kinds can injure the heart muscle. In probably nearly every case of diphtheria, unless of the mildest type, there is some myocardial involvement, even if not more than 25 percent of such cases show clinical symptoms of such heart injury. Tuberculosis of different parts of the body also, sooner or later, injures the heart; and the effect of syphilis on the heart is now well recognized.

SYMPTOMS AND SIGNS OF CARDIAC DISTURBANCE

It is now recognized that any infection can cause weakness and degeneration of the heart muscle. The Streptococcus rheumaticus found in rheumatic joints is probably the cause of such heart injury in rheumatism. That prolonged fever from any cause injures heart muscle has long been recognized, and cardiac dilatation after severe illness is now more carefully prevented. It is not sufficiently recognized that chronic, slow-going infection can injure the heart. Such infections most frequently occur in the tonsils, in the gums, and in the sinuses around the nose. Tonsillitis, acute or chronic, has been shown to be a menace to the heart. Acute streptococcie tonsillitis is a very frequent disease, and the patient generally, under proper treatment, quickly recovers. Tonsillitis in a more or less acute form, however, sometimes so mild as to be almost unnoticed, probably precedes most attacks of acute inflammatory rheumatism. Chronically diseased tonsils may not cause joint pains or acute fever, but they are certainly often the source of blood infection and later of cardiac inflammations. The probability of chronic inflammation and weakening of the heart muscle from such slow-going and continuous infection must be recognized, and the source of such infection removed.

The determination of the presence of valvular lesions is only a small part of the physical examination of the heart. Furthermore, the heart is too readily eliminated from the cause of the general disturbance because murmurs are not heard. A careful decision as to the size of the heart will often show that it has become slightly dilated and is a cause of the general symptoms of weakness, leg weariness, slight dyspnea, epigastric distress or actual chest pains. Many such cases are treated for gastric disturbance because there are some gastric symptoms. There is no question that gastric flatulence, or hyperacidity, or a large meal causing distention of the stomach may increase the cardiac disturbance, and the cardiac disturbance may be laid entirely to indigestion; but treatment directed toward the stomach, while it may ameliorate some of the symptoms, will not remove the cause of the symptoms.

If the patient complains of pains in any part of the chest or upper abdomen, or of leg aches, or of being weary, or exhausted, or of sleeplessness at night, or of pains in the back of his head, we should investigate the cardiac ability, besides ruling out all of the more frequently recognized causes of these disturbances.

If there is more dyspnea than normally should occur in the individual patient after walking rapidly or climbing a hill or going upstairs, or if after a period of a little excitement one finds that he cannot breathe quite normally, or that something feels tight in his chest, the heart needs resting. If, after one has been driving a motor car or even sitting at rest in one which has been going at speed or has come unpleasantly near to hitting something or to being run into, it is noticed that the little period of cardiac disturbance and chest tension is greater than it should be, the heart needs resting.

If the least excitement or exertion increases the cardiac speed abnormally, it means that for many minutes, if not actually hours during the twenty-four, the heart is contracting too rapidly, and this alone means muscle tire and muscle nutrition lost, even if there is no actual defect in the cardiac muscle or in its own blood supply. If we multiply these extra pulsations or contractions by the number of minutes a day that this extra amount of work is done, it will easily be demonstrable to the physician and the patient what an amount of good a rest, however partial, each twenty-four hours will do to this heart. Of course anything that tends to increase the activity of the disturbance of the heart should be corrected. Overeating, overdrinking (even water), and overuse or perhaps any use of alcohol, tobacco, tea and coffee should all be prevented. In fact, we come right to the discussion of the proper treatment and management of beginning high blood pressure, of the incipiency of arteriosclerosis, of the prevention of chronic interstitial nephritis, and the prevention of cardiovascular-renal disease.

When an otherwise apparently well person begins to complain of weariness, or perhaps drowsiness in the daytime and sleeplessness at night, or his sleep is disturbed, or be has feelings of mental depression, or he says that he "senses" his heart, perhaps for the first time in his life, with or without edema of the feet and legs, or pains referred to the heart or heart region, we should presuppose that there is weakening of the heart muscle until, by perfect examination, we have excluded the heart as being the cause of such disturbance.

Although constantly repeated by all books on the heart and by many articles on cardiac pain, it still is often forgotten that pain due to cardiac disturbance may be referred to the shoulders, to the upper part of the chest, to the axillae, to the arms, and even to the wrists, to the neck, into the head, and into the upper abdomen. It is perhaps generally auricular disturbance that causes pain to ascend, but disturbances of the ventricles can cause pain in the arms and in the region of the stomach. Not infrequently disturbances of the aorta cause pain over the right side of the chest as well as tip into the neck. Real heart pains frequently occur without any valvular lesion, and also when necropsies have shown that there has been no sclerosis of the coronary vessels.

While angina pectoris is a distinct, well recognized condition, pains in the regions mentioned, especially if they occur after exertion or after mental excitement or even after eating (provided a real gastric excuse has been eliminated), are due to a disturbance of the heart, generally to an overstrained heart muscle or to a slight dilatation. Too much or too little blood in the cavity of the heart may cause distress and pain; or an imperfect circulation through the coronary arteries and the vessels of the heart, impairing its nutrition or causing it to tire more readily, may be the cause of these cardiac pains, distress or discomfort.

Palpating the radial artery is not absolutely reliable in all cases of auricular fibrillation, or in another form of arrhythmia called auricular flutter or tachysystole. James and Hart [Footnote: James and Hart: Am. Jour. Med. Sc., 1914, cxlvii, 63.] have found that the pulse is not a true criterion of the condition Of the circulation. There is always a certain amount of heart block associated with auricular fibrillation so that not all of the auricular stimuli pass through the bundle of His. James and Hart determine the heart rate both at the radial pulse and at the apex, the difference being called the pulse deficit. They use this deficit as an aid in deciding when to stop the administration of digitalis. When the pulse deficit is zero, the digitalis is stopped. In this connection they also find that, even though the pulse deficit may be zero, there may be a difference in force and size of the waves at the radial artery. This can be demonstrated by the use of a cuff around the brachial artery and by varying the pressure. It will be found that the greater the pressure, the fewer the number of beats coming through.

Besides the instruments of precision referred to above, more careful percussion, more careful auscultation, more careful measurements, roentgenoscopy and fluoroscopic examination of the heart, and a study of the circulation with the patient standing, sitting, lying and after exercise make the determination of circulatory ability a specialty, and the physician who becomes an expert a specialist. It is a specialization needed today almost more than in any other line of medical science.

So frequently is the cause of these pains, disturbances and weakness overlooked and the stomach or the intestines treated, or treatment aimed at neuralgias, rheumatisms or rheumatic conditions, that a careful examination of the patient, and a consideration of the part the heart is playing in the causation of these symptoms are always necessary.

The treatment required for such a heart, unless there is some complication, as a kidney complication or a too high blood pressure, or arteriosclerosis (and none of these causes necessarily prohibits energetic cardiac treatment), is digitalis. If there is doubt as to the condition of the cardiac arteries, digitalis should be given in small doses. If it causes distinct cardiac pain, it is not indicated and should be stopped. If, on the other hand, improvement occurs, as it generally does, the dose can be regulated by the results. The minimum dose which improves the condition is the proper one. Enough should be given; too much should not be given. Before deciding that digitalis does not improve the condition (provided it does not cause cardiac pain) the physician should know that a good and efficient preparation of digitalis is being taken. Strychnin will sometimes whip up a tired heart and tide it over periods of depression, but it is a whip and not a cardiac tonic. While overeating, all overexertion, and alcohol should be stopped, and the amount of tobacco should be modified, there is no treatment so successful as mental and physical rest and a change of climate and scene, with good clean air.

Many persons with these symptoms of cardiac tire think that they are house-tired, shop-tired, or office-tired, and take on a physical exercise, such as walking, climbing, tennis playing or golf playing, to their injury. Such tired hearts are not ready yet for added physical exercise; they should be rested first.

The treatment of this cardiac tire is not complete until the tonsils, gums, teeth and the nose and its accessory sinuses are in good condition. Various other sources of chronic poisoning from chronic infection should of course be eliminated, whether an uncured gonorrhea, prostatitis, some chronic inflammation of the female pelvic organs, or a chronic appendicitis.

Longcope [Footnote: Longcope, W. T.: The Effect of Repeated Injections of Foreign Protein on the Heart Muscle, Arch. Int. Med., June, 1915, p. 1079.] has recently shown that repeated, and even at times one protein poisoning can cause degeneration of the heart muscle in rabbits. Hence it is quite possible that repeated absorption of protein poisons from the intestines may injure the heart muscle as well as the kidney structure; consequently, in heart weakness, besides removing all evident sources of infection, we should also give such food and cause such intestinal activity as to preclude the absorption of protein poison from the bowels.

CLASSIFICATION OF CARDIAC DISTURBANCES

For the sake of discussing the therapy of cardiac disturbances in a logical sequence, they may be classified as follows:

- Pericarditis
  - Acute
  - Adherent

- Myocarditis
  - Acute
  - Chronic
  - Fatty

- Endocarditis
  - Acute, simple malignant
  - Chronic
- Valvular Lesions
  - Broken compensation
  - Cardiac drugs
  - Diet
  - Resort treatment
- Cardiac disease in children
- Cardiac disease in pregnancy
- Coronary sclerosis
- Angina pectoris
  - Pseudo-angina
- Stokes-Adams disease
- Arterial hypertension
- Cardiovascular-renal disease
- Arrhythmia
- Auricular fibrillation
- Bradycardia
- Paroxysmal tachycardia

Hyperthyroidism
Toxic disturbances
Physiologic hypertrophies
Simple dilatation
Shock
Stomach dilatation
Anesthesia in heart disease

BLOOD PRESSURE

The study of the blood pressure has become a subject of great importance in the practice of medicine and surgery. No condition can be properly treated, no operation should be performed, and no prognosis is of value without a proper consideration of the sufficiency of the circulation, and the condition of the circulation cannot be properly estimated without an accurate estimate of the systolic and diastolic blood pressure. However perfectly the heart may act, it cannot properly circulate the blood without a normal tone of the blood vessels, both arteries and veins. Abnormal vasodilatation seriously interferes with the normal circulation, and causes venous congestion, abnormal increase in venous blood pressure, and the consequent danger of shock and death. Increased arterial tone or tonicity necessitates greater cardiac effort, to overcome the resistance, and hypertrophy of the heart must follow. This hypertrophy always occurs if the peripheral resistance is not suddenly too great or too rapidly acquired. In other words, if the peripheral resistance gradually increases, the left ventricle hypertrophies, and remains for a long time sufficient. If, from disease or disturbance in the lungs, the resistance in the pulmonary circulation is increased, the right ventricle hypertrophies to overcome it, and the circulation is sufficient as long as this ventricle is able to do the work. If either this pulmonary increased pressure or the systemic increased pressure persists or becomes too great, it is only a question of how many months, in the case of the right ventricle, and how many years, in the case of the left ventricle, the heart can stand the strain.

If the cause of the increased systemic tension is an arterial fibrosis, sooner or later the heart will become involved in this general condition, and a chronic myocarditis is likely to result. If, on the other hand, there is a continuous low systemic arterial blood pressure, the circulation is always more or less insufficient, nutrition is always imperfect, and the physical ability of the individual is below par. It is evident, therefore, that an abnormally high blood pressure is of serious import, its cause must be studied, and effort must be made to remove as far as possible the cause. On the other hand, a persistently low blood pressure may be of serious import, and always diminishes physical ability. If possible, the cause should be determined, and the condition improved.

No physician can now properly practice medicine without having a reliable apparatus for determining the blood pressure both in his office and at the bedside. It is not necessary to discuss here the various kinds of apparatus or what is essential in an apparatus for it to give a perfect reading. It may be stated that in determining the systolic and diastolic pressure in the peripheral arteries, the ordinary stethoscope is as efficient as any more elaborate auscultatory apparatus.

It is now generally agreed by all scientific clinicians that it is as essential—almost more essential—to determine the diastolic pressure as the systolic pressure; therefore the auscultatory method is the simplest, as well as one of the most accurate in determining these pressures. Of course it should be recognized that the systolic pressure thus obtained will generally be some millimeters above that obtained with the finger, perhaps the average being equivalent to about 5 mm. of mercury. The diastolic pressure will often range from 10 to 15 mm. below the reading obtained by other methods. Therefore, wider range of pressure is obtained by the auscultatory method than by other methods. This difference of 5 or more millimeters of systolic pressure between the auscultatory and the palpatory readings should be remembered when one is consulting books or articles printed more than two years ago, as many of these pressures were determined by the palpatory method.

Sometimes the compression of the arm by the armlet leads to a rise in blood pressure. [Footnote: MacWilliams and Melvin: Brit. Med. Jour., Nov. 7, 1914.] It has been suggested that the diastolic pressure be taken at the point where the sound is first heard on gradually raising the pressure in the armlet.

In some persons the auscultatory readings cannot be made, or are very unsatisfactory, and it becomes necessary to use the palpation method in taking the systolic pressure. In instances in which the auscultatory method is unsatisfactory, the artery below the bend of the elbow at which the reading is generally taken may be misplaced, or there may be an unusual amount of fat and muscle between the artery and the skin.

The various sounds heard with the stethoscope, when the pressure is gradually lowered, have been divided into phases. The first phase begins with the first audible sound, which is the proper point at which to read the, systolic pressure. The first phase is generally, not always, succeeded by a second phase in which there is a murmurish sound. The third phase is that at which the maximum sharp, ringing note begins, and throughout this phase the sound is sharp and intense, gradually increasing, and then gradually diminishing to the fourth phase, where the sound suddenly becomes a duller tone. The fourth phase lasts until what is termed the fifth phase, or that at which all sound has disappeared. As previously stated, the diastolic pressure may be read at the beginning of the fourth phase, or at the end of the fourth phase, that is, the beginning of the fifth; but the difference is from 3 to 10 mm. of mercury, with an average of perhaps 5 mm.; therefore the difference is not very great. When the diastolic pressure is high, for relative subsequent readings, it is much better to read the diastolic at the beginning of the fifth phase.

It is urged by many observers that the proper reading of the diastolic pressure is always at the beginning of the fourth phase. However, for general use, unless one is particularly expert, it is better to read the diastolic pressure at the beginning of the fifth phase. There can rarely be a doubt in the mind of the person who is auscultating as to the point at which all sound ceases. There is frequently a good deal of doubt, even after large experience, as to just the moment at which the fourth phase begins. With the understanding that the difference is only a few millimeters, which is of very little importance, when the diastolic pressure is below 95, it seems advisable to urge the reading of the diastolic pressure at the beginning of the fifth phase.

The incident of the first phase, or when sound begins, is caused by the sudden distention of the blood vessel below the point of compression by the armlet. In other words, the armlet pressure has at this point been overcome. Young [Footnote: Young: Indiana State Med. Assn. Jour., March, 1914.] believes that the murmurs of the second phase, which in all normal conditions are heard during the 20 mm. drop below the point at which the systolic pressure had been read, is "due to whirlpool eddies produced at the point of constriction of the blood vessel by the cuff of the instrument." The third phase is when these murmurs cease and the sound resembles the first, lasting he thinks for only 5 mm. The third phase often lasts much longer. He thinks the fourth phase, when the sound becomes dull, lasts for about 6 mm.

TECHNIC

It is essential that the patient on whom the examination is to be made should be at rest, either comfortably seated, or lying down. All clothing should be removed from the arm, and there should be no constriction by sleeves, either of the upper arm or the axilla. When the blood pressure is taken over the sleeve of a garment, the instrument will register from 10 to 30 mm. higher than on the bare arm. [Footnote: Rowan, J. J.: The Practical Application of Blood Pressure Findings, The JOURNAL A. M. A., March 18, 1916, p. 873.]

While it may be better, for insurance examinations, to take the blood pressure of the left arm in right handed persons as a truer indicator of the general condition, the difference is generally not great. The right arm of right handed persons usually registers a full 5 mm. higher systolic pressure than the left arm.

The patient, being at rest and removed as far as possible from all excitement, may be conversed with to take his mind away from the fact that his blood pressure is being taken. He also should not watch the dial, as any tensity on his part more or less raises the systolic pressure, the diastolic not being much affected by such nervous tension. The armlet having been carefully applied, it is better to inflate gradually 10 mm. higher than the point at which the pulsation ceases in the radial. The stethoscope is then firmly applied, but with not too great pressure, to the forearm just below the flexure of the elbow. The exact point at which the sound is heard in the individual patient, and the exact amount of pressure that must be applied, will be determined by the first reading, and then thus applied to the second reading. One reading is never sufficient for obtaining the correct blood pressure. The blood pressure may be read by means of the stethoscope during the gradual raising of pressure in the cuff, note being taken of the first sound that is heard (the diastolic pressure), and the point at which all sound disappears, as the pressure is increased (the systolic pressure). The former method is the one most frequently used.

By taking the systolic and diastolic pressures, the difference between the two being the pressure pulse, we learn to interpret the pressure pulse reading. While the average pressure pulse has frequently been stated as 30 mm., it is probable that 35 at least, and often 40 mm. represents more nearly the normal pressure pulse, and from 25 mm. on the one hand to 50 on the other may not be abnormal.

Faught [Footnote: Faught: New York Med Jour., Feb. 27, 1915, p. 396.] states his belief that the relation of the pressure pulse to the diastolic pressure and the systolic pressure are as 1, 2 and 3. In other words, a normal young adult with a systolic pressure of 120 should have a diastolic pressure of 80, and therefore a pulse pressure of 40. If these relationships become much abnormal, disease is developing and imperfect circulation is in evidence, with the danger of broken compensation occurring at some time in the future.

It should be remembered that the diastolic pressure represents the pressure which the left ventricle must overcome before the blood will begin to circulate, that is, before the aortic valve opens, while the pressure pulse represents the power of the left ventricle in excess of the diastolic pressure. Therefore it is easy to understand that a high diastolic pressure is of serious import to the heart; a diastolic pressure over 100 is significant of trouble, and over 110 is a menace.

FACTORS INCREASING THE BLOOD PRESSURE

With normal heart and arteries, exertion and exercise should increase the systolic pressure, and generally somewhat increase the diastolic pressure. The pressure pulse should therefore be greater. When there is circulatory defect or abnormal blood pressure, exercise may not increase the systolic pressure, and the pressure pulse may grow smaller. As a working rule it should be noted that the diastolic pressure is not as much influenced by physiologic factors or the varying conditions of normal life as is the systolic pressure.

In an irregularly acting heart the systolic pressure may vary greatly, from 10 to 20 mm. or more, and a ventricular contraction may not be of sufficient power to open the semilunar valves. Such beats will show an intermittency in the blood pressure reading as well as in the radial pulse. The succeeding heart beats after abortive beats or after a contraction of less power have increased force, and consequently give the highest blood pressure. Kilgore urges that these highest pressures should not be taken as the true systolic blood pressure, but the average of a series of these varying blood pressures. In irregularly acting hearts it is best to compress the arm at a point above which the systolic pressure is heard, then gradually reduce the pressure until the first systolic pressure is recorded, and then keep the pressure of the cuff at this point and record the number of beats of the heart which are heard during the minute. Then reduce the pressure 5 mm. and read again for a minute, and so on down the scale until the varying systolic pressures are recorded. The average of these pressures should be read as the true systolic blood pressure. During an intermittency of the pulse from a weak or intermittently acting ventricle, the diastolic pressure will reach its lowest point, and in auricular fibrillation the pressure pulse from the highest systolic to the lowest diastolic may be very great.

In arteriosclerosis the systolic may be high, and the diastolic low, and hence a large pressure pulse. When the heart begins to fail in this condition, the systolic pressure drops and the pressure pulse shortens, and of course any improvement in this condition will be shown by an increase in the systolic pressure. The same is true with aortic regurgitation and a high systolic pressure.

If the systolic pressure is low and the diastolic very low, or when the heart is rapid, circulation through the coronary vessels of the heart is more or less imperfect. Any increase in arterial pressure will therefore help the coronary circulation. The compression of a tight bandage around the abdomen, or the infusion of blood or saline solutions, especially when combined with minute amounts of epinephrin, will raise the blood pressure and increase the coronary circulation and therefore the nutrition of the heart.

MacKenzie [Footnote: MacKenzie: Med Rec., New York, Dec. 18, 1915.], from a large number of insurance examinations in normal subjects, finds that for each increase of 5 pulse beats the pressure rises 1 mm. He also finds that the effect of height on blood pressure in adults seems to be negligible. On the other hand, it is now generally proved that persons with overweight have a systolic pressure greater than is normal for individuals of the same age. He believes that diastolic pressure may range anywhere from 60 mm. of mercury to 105, and the person still be normal. A figure much below 60 certainly shows dangerous loss of pressure, and one far below this, except in profound heart weakness, is almost pathognomonic of aortic regurgitation. While the systolic range from youth to over 60 years of age gradually increases, at the younger age anything below 105 mm. of mercury should be considered abnormally low, and although 150 mm. at anything over 40 has been considered a safe blood pressure as long as the diastolic was below 105, such pressures are certainly a subject for investigation, and if the systolic pressure is persistently above 150, insurance companies dislike to take the risk. However, it should be again urged in making insurance examinations that psychic disturbance or mental tensity very readily raises the systolic pressure. MacKenzie believes that a diastolic pressure over 100 under the age of 40 is abnormal, and anything over the 110 mark above that age is certainly abnormal.

It has been shown, notably by Barach and Marks, [Footnote: Barach, J. H., and Marks, W. L.: Effect of Change of Posture—Without Active Muscular Exertion—on the Arterial and Venous Pressures, Arch. Int. Med., May, 1913, p 485.] that posture changes the blood pressure. When a normal person reclines, with the muscular system relaxed, there is an increase in the systolic pressure and a decrease in the diastolic pressure, with an increase in the pressure pulse from the figures found when the person is standing. When, after some minutes of repose, he assumes the erect posture again, the systolic pressure will diminish and the diastolic pressure increase, and the pressure pulse shortens.

Excitement can raise the blood pressure from 20 to 30 mm., and if such excitement occurs in high tension cases there is often a systolic blow in the second intercostal space at the right of the sternum. This may not be due to narrowing of the aortic orifice; it may be due to a sclerosis of the aorta. On the other hand, it may be due entirely to the hastened blood stream from the nervous excitability. This is probably the case if this sound disappears when the patient reclines. If it increases when the heart becomes slower and the patient is lying down, the cause is probably organic.

This psychic influence on blood pressure is stated by Maloney and Sorapure [Footnote: Maloney and Sorapure: New York Med. Jour., May 23, 1914, p. 1021.] "to be greater than that from posture, than that arising from carbonic acid gas control of the blood, than that arising from mechanical action of deep breathing upon the circulation, and than that arising from removal of spasm from the musculature."

Weysse and Lutz [Footnote: Weysse and Lutz: Am. Jour. Physiol., May, 1915.] find that the systolic pressure varies during the day in normal persons, and is increased by the taking of food, on an average of 8 mm. The diastolic pressure is not much affected by food. This increased systolic pressure is the greatest about half an hour after a meal, and then gradually declines until the next meal.

Any active, hustling man, or a man under strain, has a rise of blood pressure during that strain, especially notable with surgeons during operation, or with brokers or persons under high nervous tension. Daland [Footnote: Daland: Pennsylvania Med Jour., July, 1913.] states that a man driving an automobile through a crowded street may have an increase of systolic pressure of 30 mm., and an increase of 15 mm. in his diastolic pressure, while the same man driving through the country where there is little traffic will increase but 10 mm. systolic and 5 mm. diastolic. Fear always increases the blood pressure. This is probably largely due to the peripheral contractions of the blood vessels and nervous chilling of the body.

VENOUS PRESSURE

The venous pressure, after a long neglect, is now again being studied, and its determination is urged as of diagnostic and prognostic significance.

Hooker [Footnote: Hooker: Am. Jour. Physiol., March, 1916.] says there is a progressive rise of venous pressure from youth to old age. He has described an apparatus [Footnote: Hooker: Am. Jour. Physiol., 1914, xxxv, 73.] which allows of the reading of the blood pressure in a vein of the hand when the arm is at absolute rest, and best with the patient in bed and reclining at an angle of 45 degrees. He finds that just before death there is a rapid rise in venous pressure, or a continuously high pressure above the 20 cm. of water level, and he believes that a venous pressure continuously above this 20 cm. of water limit which is not lowered by digitalis or other means is serious; and that the heart cannot long stand such a condition. These dangerous rises in venous pressure are generally coincident with a fall of systolic arterial pressure, although there may be no constant relation between the two. He also finds that with an increase of venous pressure the urinary output decreases. This, of course, shows venous stasis in the kidneys as well as a probable lowering of arterial pressure.

Clark [Footnote: Clark, A. D.: A Study of the Diagnostic and Prognostic Significance of Venous Pressure Observations in Cardiac Disease, Arch. Int. Med., October, 1915, p. 587.] did not find that venesection prevented a subsequent rapid rise in venous pressure in dire cases. From his investigations he concludes that a venous pressure of 20 cm. of water is a danger limit between compensation and decompensation of the heart, and a rise above this point will precede the clinical signs of decompensation.

Hooker also found that there are daily variations of venous pressure from 10 to 20 cm. of water, with an average of 15 cm., while in sleep it falls 7 or 8 cm.

It seems probable that there may be a special nervous mechanism of the veins which may increase the blood pressure in them as epinephrin solution may cause some constriction.

Wiggers [Footnote: Wiggers C. J.: The Supravascular Venous Pulse in Man, THE JOURNAL. A.M.A., May 1, 1915, p. 1485.] describes a method of taking and interpreting the supraclavicular venous pulse. He also [Footnote: Wiggers C. J.: The Contour of the Normal Arterial Pulse, THE JOURNAL. A.M.A., April 24, 1915, p. 1380.] carefully describes the readings and the different phases of normal arterial pulse, and urges that it should be remembered that "the pulse as palpated or recorded from any artery is the variation in the arterial volume produced by the intra-arterial pressure change at that point."

A quick method of estimating the venous pressure by lowering and raising the arm has long been utilized. The dilatation of the veins of the back of the hand when the hand is raised should disappear, and they should practically collapse, in normal conditions, when the hand is at the level of the apex of the heart. When the venous pressure is increased, this collapse will not occur until the hand is above the level of the heart. Oliver [Footnote: Oliver: Quart. Med Jour., 1907, i, 59.] found that the venous pressure denoted by the collapse of the veins may be shown approximately in millimeters of mercury by multiplying by 2 each inch above the level of the heart in which the veins collapse. When a normal person reclines after standing there is a fall in venous pressure, and when he again stands erect there is an increase in venous pressure.

Bailey [Footnote: Bailey: Am. Jour Med. Sc., May, 1911, p. 709.] states that in interpreting pulsation in the peripheral veins, it should not be forgotten that they may overlie pulsating arteries. Pulsation in veins may be due also to an aneurysmal dilatation, or to direct connection with an artery. As the etiology in many instances of varicose veins is uncertain, he thinks that they may be caused by incompetence of the right heart, more or less temporary perhaps, from muscular exertion. This incompetence being frequently repeated, peripheral veins may dilate. Moreover, the contraction of the right heart may cause a wave in the veins of the extremities, and he believes that incompetency of the tricuspid valve may be the cause of varicosities in the veins of the extremities.

NORMAL BLOOD PRESSURE FOR ADULTS

Woley [Footnote: Woley, II. P.: The Normal Variation of the Systolic Blood Pressure, THE JOURNAL A. M. A., July 9, 1910, p. 121.] after studying, the blood pressure in a thousand persons, found that the systolic average for males at all ages was 127.5 mm., while that for females at all ages was 120 mm. He found the average in persons from 15 to 30 years to be 122 systolic; from 30 to 40, 127 mm., and from the ages of 40 to 50, to be 130 mm.

Lee [Footnote: Lee: Boston Med. and Surg. Jour., Oct. 7, 1915.] examined 662 young men at the average age of 18, and found that the average systolic blood pressure was 120 mm., and the average diastolic 80 mm. Eighty-five of these young men, however, had a systolic pressure of over 140. It is not unusual to find that a young man who is very athletic has an abnormally high systolic pressure.

Barach and Marks [Footnote: Barach, J. H., and Marks, W. L.: Blood Pressures: Their Relation to Each Other and to Physical Efficiency, Arch. Int. Med., April, 1914, p 648.] in a series of 656 healthy young men, found that the systolic pressure was above 150 in only 10 percent, and that in 338 cases the diastolic pressure, read at the fifth phase, did not exceed 100 mm. in 96 percent

Nicholson [Footnote: Nicholson: Am. Jour. Med. Sc., April, 1914, p. 514.] believes that with a low systolic pressure and a large pressure pulse there is probably a strong heart and dilated blood vessels, while with a low systolic pressure and a small pressure pulse the heart itself is weak, with also, perhaps, dilated blood vessels. If there is a high systolic pressure and a correspondingly high diastolic pressure, the balance between the vessels and the heart is compensated as long as the heart muscle is sufficient. He believes the velocity of the blood in the blood stream may be roughly estimated as being equal to the pressure pulse multiplied by the pulse rate.

Faber 44 [Footnote: Faber: Ugeskrifta f. Laeger, June 10, 1915.] examined 211 obese patients, and in 182 of these there was no kidney or vascular disturbance. In 52 percent of these 211 persons the systolic pressure was under 140, while in the remaining 48 percent it ranged from 145 to 200 mm.

BLOOD PRESSURE IN CHILDREN

May Michael, [Footnote: Michael, May: A Study of Blood Pressure in Normal Children, Am. Jour. Dis. Child., April, 1911, p. 272.] after a study of the blood pressure in 350 children, came to the conclusion that the blood pressure in children increases with age principally because of the increase in height and weight, as she found that children of the same age but of different weights and heights had different blood pressures. Sex in children makes no difference in the blood pressure, it being determined by the height and weight.

Judson and Nicholson [Footnote: Judson, C. F., and Nicholson, Percival: Blood Pressure in Normal Children, Am. Jour. Dis. Child., October, 1914, p. 257.] made 2,300 observations in children of from 3 to 15 years of age, and found there was a gradual increase in the systolic blood pressure from 3 to 10 years, and a more rapid rise from 10 to 14, with a rapid elevation during the fourteenth year, or the age of puberty. The systolic pressure varied from 91 mm. in the fourth year to 105.5 in the fourteenth year, while the diastolic pressure remained almost at a uniform level. The pressure pulse, therefore, increased progressively with the increase of the systolic pressure.

BLOOD PRESSURE AND INSURANCE

An epitome of the consensus of opinion of the risk of accepting persons for insurance as modified by the blood pressure is presented by Quackenbos. [Footnote: Quackenbos: New York Med. Jour., May 15, 1915, p. 999.] Some companies have ruled that at the age of 20 they will take a person with a systolic pressure up to 137; at the age of 30 up to 140; at the age of 40 up to 144; at 50 up to 148, and at 60 up to 153, although some companies will not accept a person who shows a persistent systolic pressure of 150. Quackenbos says that when persons with higher blood pressures than the foregoing have been kept under observation for some time, they sooner or later show albumin and casts in the urine. In other words, this stage of higher blood pressure is too frequently followed by cardiovascular-renal disease for insurance companies to accept the risk.

On the other hand, too low a systolic pressure in an adult, 105 mm. or below, should cause suspicion of some serious condition, the most frequent being a latent or quiescent tuberculosis. Such low pressure certainly shows decreased power of resistance to any acute disease.

Statistics prove that there are more deaths between the ages of 40 and 50 from cardiovascular-renal disease, that is from heart, arterial and kidney degenerations, than formerly. Whether this is due to the high tension at which we all live, or to the fact that more children are saved and live to middle life, or whether the prevention of many infectious diseases saves deficient individuals for this middle life period, has not been determined. Probably all are factors in bringing about these statistics.

While the continued use of alcohol may not cause arteriosclerosis directly, it can cause such impaired digestion of foods in the stomach and intestine, and such impaired activity of the glands, especially the liver, that toxins from imperfect digestion and from waste products are more readily produced and absorbed, and these are believed by some directly or indirectly to cause cardiovascular-renal disease. Hence alcohol is an important factor in causing the death of persons from 40 to 50 years of age.

The question of whether or not a person smokes too much, and what constitutes oversmoking, will soon be asked on all insurance blanks. As tobacco almost invariably raises the blood pressure, and when the blood pressure again falls there is again a craving in the man for the narcotic, it must be a factor in producing, later in life, cardiovascular-renal disease. Hence an increased systolic blood pressure must be in part interpreted by the amount of tobacco that the person uses. BLOOD PRESSURE AND PREGNANCY Evans [Footnote: Evans: Month. Cyc. and Med. Bull., November, 1912, p. 649.] of Montreal studied thirty-eight pregnant women who had eclampsia, albuminuria and toxic vomiting, and found the systolic pressures to vary from 200 to 140 mm. He did not find that the highest pressures necessarily showed the greatest insufficiency of the kidneys, but that the blood pressure must be considered in conjunction with other toxic symptoms. In thirty-two cases he was compelled to induce labor when the blood pressure was 150 mm. or under, while in four cases with a blood pressure over 150 mm., the toxic symptoms were so slight that the patients were allowed to go to term and had natural deliveries.

A rising blood pressure in pregnancy, when associated with other toxic symptoms, is indicative of danger, and Evans believes that a systolic pressure of 160 mm, is ordinarily the danger limit.

Newell [Footnote: Newell, h. S.: The Blood Pressure During Pregnancy, THE JOURNAL A. M. A., Jan. 30, 1915, p. 393.] has studied the blood pressure during normal pregnancy, and finds that when the systolic pressure is persistently below 100, the patient is far below par, and that the condition should be improved in order for her to withstand the strain of parturition. When the systolic pressure is above 130, the patient should be carefully watched, and he thinks that 150 is the danger line. Some pregnant women have an increasing rise in blood pressure throughout the pregnancy, without albuminuria. In other cases this rise is followed by the appearance of albumin in the urine. Thirty-nine of the patients studied by Newell had albumin in the urine without increase in blood pressure; hence he believes that a slight amount of albumin may not be accompanied by other symptoms. Five patients had a blood pressure of 140 or over throughout their pregnancy, and in only one of these patients was albumin found. All passed through labor normally, showing that a blood pressure below 150 may not necessarily be indicative of a serious condition; but a patient who has a systolic pressure over 135 must certainly be carefully watched. A fact brought out by Newell's investigations is very important, namely, that a continuously increased blood pressure is not as indicative of trouble as when a blood pressure has been low and later suddenly rises.

Hirst [Footnote: Hirst: Pennsylvania Med. Jour., May, 1915, p. 615.] also urges that a high blood pressure in pregnancy does not necessarily represent a toxemia, and also that a serious toxemia can occur with a blood pressure of 130 or lower, although such instances are rare. Hirst believes that when a toxemia is in evidence in pregnancy while the blood pressure is low, the cause of the toxemia is liver disturbance rather than kidney disturbance, and he thinks this form of toxemia is more serious and has a higher mortality than the nephritic type. Therefore in a patient with eclamptic symptoms and a low blood pressure, the prognosis is more unfavorable than when the blood pressure is high. He believes that if high blood pressure occurs early in the months of pregnancy, there is preexisting, although perhaps latent, nephritis. In these conditions the diastolic pressure is also likely to be high.

With the patient eclamptic and stupid, whatever the date of the pregnancy, Hirst would do venesection immediately in amount from 16 to 24 ounces, depending on what amount seems advisable. If venesection is done before actual convulsions have occurred, the blood pressure falls temporarily but rapidly rises again. He finds that if a patient is past the eighth month, rupture of the membranes will usually bring a rapid fall of from 50 to 90 points in systolic pressure. Usually, of course, such rupture of the membranes will induce labor. He finds that the fluidextract of veratrum viride is valuable when eclampsia is in evidence or imminent. He gives it hypodermically, 15 minims at the first dose and 5 minims subsequently, until the systolic pressure is reduced to 140 or less. He admits that this is rather strenuous treatment. He does not speak of treatment by thyroid extracts, which has been regarded as valuable by some other workers.

In these patients who show eclamptic symptoms, he maintains a milk diet, and purging and sweating. It should be remembered that venesection or profuse bleeding during induced parturition is more valuable than sweating in all eclamptic cases and in all nephritic convulsions. Profuse sweating does little more than take the water out of the blood, and even concentrates the poisons in the blood.

Hirst causes purging by 2 ounces of castor oil and a few minims of croton oil. He also advises large doses of magnesium sulphate. In such serious disturbances as eclampsia, it is not necessary to give a magnesium salt, which, it has been shown, can have unpleasant action on the nervous system. Sodium sulphate is as valuable and is not open to this danger.

Hirst urges that whatever the blood pressure, with albuminuria, as soon as persistent headache occurs, and especially if there are disturbances of vision, the pregnancy must be terminated at once.

On this there can be no other opinion. Temporizing with such a case is inexcusable.

After labor has been induced there is an immediate fall of blood pressure, which lasts some hours. The pressure will again rise, and usually is the last sign of toxemia to disappear, and he finds that this increased pressure may last from two to three weeks when there is not much nephritis, and several months when there is nephritis.

Although he says he has found no bad action from ergot, either by the mouth or hypodermically in these eclamptic cases, it would seem inadvisable to use ergot, which may raise the blood pressure. He finds that pituitary extract "can cause dangerous rise of blood pressure."

Pelissier [Footnote: Pelissier: Archiv. mens., d'obst. et de gynec., Paris, 1915, iv, No. 5.] believes that when there is prolonged vomiting in early pregnancy, with an increase in systolic blood pressure, and with an increased viscosity of the blood, the outlook is serious, and active treatment should be inaugurated.

Irving [Footnote: Irving, F. C.: The Systolic Blood Pressure in Pregnancy, THE JOURNAL A. M. A., March 25, 1916, p. 935.] reports, after a study of 5,000 pregnant women, that in 80 percent the systolic blood pressure varied from 100 to 130; in 9 percent it was below 100, at least at times, but a pressure below 90 does not mean that the woman will suffer shock; in 11 percent the pressure was above 130, and high pressure in young pregnant women more frequently indicates toxemia than when it occurs in older women; high pressure is more indicative of toxemia than is albuminuria; a progressively increasing blood pressure is of bad omen, and most cases of eclampsia occur with a pressure of 160 or more, but eclampsia may occur with a moderate blood pressure. Irving believes that with proper preliminary preventive treatment most eclampsia is preventable.

ALTITUDE

It has long been known that altitude increases the heart rate and tends to lower the systolic and diastolic blood pressures; that these conditions, though actively present at first, gradually return to normal, and that after a prolonged stay at the altitude may become nearly normal for the individual. Burker [Footnote: Burker, K.; Jooss, E.; Moll, E., and Neumann, E.: Ztschr. f. Biol., 1913, lxi, 379. The Influence of Altitude on the Blood, editorial, THE JOURNAL A. M. A., Nov. 1, 1913, p. 1634.] showed that altitude increases the red blood cells from 4 to 11.5 percent, and the hemoglobin from 7 to 10 percent The greatest increase in these readings is in the first few days. It has also been shown that with every 100 mm. of fall of atmospheric pressure there is an increased hemoglobin percentage of 10 percent over that at the sea level. [Footnote: Blood and Respiration at Moderate Altitudes, editorial, THE JOURNAL A. M. A., Feb. 20, 1915, p. 670.]

Schneider and Havens [Footnote: Schneider and Havens: Am. Jour. Physiol., March, 1915.] find that in low altitudes abdominal massage increases the red corpuscles, and the percentage of hemoglobin in the peripheral vessels. While there is thus apparently a reserve of red corpuscles while the individual is in a low altitude, in a high altitude they find such reserve to be absent; in other words, abdominal massage did not cause this increase in red corpuscles in the peripheral vessels. This absence of reserve is easily accounted for by the fact that after one reaches the high altitude there is an increase in red corpuscles and hemoblogin in the peripheral blood.

Schneider and Hedblom [Footnote: Schneider and Hedblom: Am. Jour., Physiol., November, 1908.] showed that the fall in systolic pressure at altitudes is greater and more certain than the fall in diastolic, some individuals even having a rise in diastolic pressure. This rise in diastolic pressure is probably caused by dyspnea.

Schrumpf, [Footnote: Schrumpf: Deutsch. Arch. f. klin. Med., 1914, cxiii, 466] on the other hand, finds that normal blood pressure is not much affected by an ascent of about 6,500 feet, while patients with arteriosclerosis and hypertension, without kidney disease, have a fall in pressure. A patient with coronary disease should certainly not go to any great altitude, while patients with compensated valvular lesions, he found, were not injured by ordinary heights. He found that altitude seemed to decrease high systolic and diastolic pressures, while it even elevated those which were below normal, and caused these patients to feel better.

Any person who has a circulatory disturbance, and who must or does go to a higher altitude, should rest for a series of days, until his blood pressure and blood have reached an equilibrium.

Smith [Footnote: Smith, F. C.: The Effect of Altitude on Blood Pressure, THE JOURNAL A. M. A., May 29, 1915, p. 1812.] made a series of observations on blood pressures at Fort Stanton which has an altitude of 6,230 feet. He took the blood pressure readings in fifty-four young adults, seventeen of whom were women, and found that the average systolic reading in the men was 129 mm., and in the women 121, while the average diastolic in the men was 84, and in the women 82. Therefore he agrees with Schrumpf that the effect of altitude on normal blood pressure has been overestimated. In tuberculosis he found that the effect of altitude was not great. He does not believe that this amount of altitude, namely, a little more than 6,000 feet, makes much difference in an ordinary tuberculous patient. He did not find that artificial pneumothorax made any important change in the blood pressure. His findings do not quite agree with Peters and Bullock, [Footnote: Peters, L. S.r and Bullock, E. S.: Blood Pressure Studies in Tuberculosis at a High Altitude, Arch. Int. Med., October, 1913, p. 456.] who studied 600 cases of tuberculosis at an altitude of 6,000 feet, and found the blood pressure was increased, both in normal and in consumptive individuals. They also found that the increase in blood pressure, which kept gradually rising up to a certain limit, was indicative that the tuberculous patient was not much toxic; therefore the increase in blood pressure was of good prognosis.

CONDITIONS CAUSING CHANGE IN BLOOD PRESSURE

Woolley [Footnote: Woolley, P. G.: Factors Governing Vascular Dilatation and Slowing of the Blood Stream in Inflammation, THE JOURNAL A. M. A., Dec. 26, 1914, p. 2279.] quotes Starling as finding that the blood vessels dilate from physical and chemical changes in the musculature, and that this dilatation is caused by deficient oxidation and accumulation of the products of metabolism, including carbon dioxid. This dilatation ordinarily is transient and not associated with exudation, but in inflammation the dilatation is persistent and there is exudation. The carbon dioxid increase during exercise stimulates a greater circulation of oxygen in the tissues which later counteracts the normal increase in acid products. In inflammatory processes, however, the acid accumulates too rapidly to allow of saturation. In this case the circulation becomes slowed and the cells become affected.

Besides these charges in the blood vessels of the muscles, the general blood pressure becomes raised on exercise, the heart more rapid and the temperature somewhat elevated, and the breathing is increased. This increased heart rate does not stop immediately on cessation of the exercise, but persists for a longer or shorter time. The better trained the individual, the sooner the speed of the heart becomes normal.

Benedict and Cathcart [Footnote: Benedict and Cathcart: Pub. 77, Carnegie Institute of Washington.] have found that the increased absorption of oxygen, showing increased metabolism, persists after exercise as long as the heart action is increased.

Newburgh and Lawrence [Footnote: Newburgh, L. H., and Lawrence C. H.: The Effect of Heat on Blood Pressure, Arch. Int. Med., February, 1914, p. 287.] have found that increased temperature in animals, equal to that occurring in persons suffering with infection, reduces the blood pressure, causing a hypotension. This shows that high temperature alone in an individual sooner or later causes hypotension.

Although prolonged pain may cause a fall of blood pressure from shock, the first acute pain may cause a rise in blood pressure, and Curschmann [Footnote: Curschmann: Munchen. med. Wehnschr., Oct. 15, 1907.] found that the blood pressure was high in the gastrointestinal crises of tabes and in colic, and that the application of faradic electricity to the thigh could raise the blood pressure from 8 to 10 mm. in normal individuals.

The positive effect of decomposition products in the intestine, more especially such as come from meat proteins, is well recognized; but the importance, in high pressure cases, of the absorption of toxins derived from imperfectly digested food remaining in the bowels over night is not sufficiently recognized. Patients with high blood pressure should not eat a heavy evening meal, and especially should they not eat meat. Willson [Footnote: Willson, R. N.: The Decomposition Food Products as Cardiovascular Products, THE JOURNAL A. M. A., Sept. 25, 1915, p. 1077.] well describes the condition caused by the absorption of these toxins. If the heart muscle is intact, he finds such absorption in high pressure cases will show diastolic as well as systolic increase:

The vessels pulsate and throb; the skin is pale; the head aches; the tongue is coated; the breath is foul; vertigo is often distressing; and not infrequently the hands and feet feel distended and swollen. A thorough house-cleaning of the gastro-intestinal canal causes the expulsion of the offending substances and the expulsion of gas, whereupon the blood pressure often resumes its normal level and the symptoms disappear.

Wilson suggests that not only the meat proteins, but also the oxyphenylethylamin in overripe cheese may often cause this poisoning; and cheese is frequently eaten by these people at bedtime. Of course if any particular fruit or article of food causes intestinal upset in a given individual, they should be avoided.

When the heart is hypertrophied in disease, the cavities of the ventricles are probably also generally enlarged, and therefore they propel more blood at each contraction than in normal persons and thus increase the blood pressure.

The blood pressure is raised not only by intestinal toxemia and uremia, but also by lead poisoning and the conditions generally present in gout.

It has been pointed out by Daland [Footnote: Daland: Pennsylvania Med. Jour., July, 1913.] that nervous exhaustion may raise the blood pressure in those who are neurotic, and he finds that this hypertension may exist for months in some cases. On the other hand, in neurasthenics the blood pressure is generally lowered. As he points out, there is often a very great increase in the systolic blood pressure at the menopause, while the diastolic pressure may not be high. This makes a very large pressure pulse. This suggests the possibility of disturbances of the glands of internal secretion. This hypertension is generally improved under proper treatment.

Schwarzmann [Footnote: Schwarzmann: Zentralbl. f. inn. Med., Aug. 1, 1914.] studied the blood pressure in eighty cases of acute infection, and found that a high diastolic blood pressure during such illness indicates a tendency to paralysis of the abdominal vessels, and hence a sluggish circulation in the vessels of the abdomen. He found that in seriously ill patients this high diastolic pressure is of bad prognosis. He also found that a lower systolic pressure with a lower diastolic pressure is not a sign that the heart is weakening, but only that the visceral tone is growing less. On the other hand, when the diastolic pressure rises while the systolic falls, this is a sign of failing heart.

Newburgh and Minot [Footnote: Newburgh, L. H. and Minot, G. II: The Blood Pressure in Pneumonia, Arch. Int. Med., July, 1914, p. 48.] find that the blood pressure course in pneumonia does not suggest that there is a failure of the vasomotor center. They found that "low systolic pressures are not invariably of evil omen." They also found that the systolic pressure in fatal cases is often higher than in those in which the patients recovered, and they found that the rate of the pulse is more important in determining the treatment than the blood pressure measurements.

The work which has been described under this section is of interest as indicating the newer experimental work on the physiology of blood pressure. Much of it is new, however, and it is difficult to draw absolute therapeutic conclusions from the evidence offered.

THE EFFECT OF DRUGS ON BLOOD PRESSURE

Free catharsis is a well established and valuable method of relieving the heart in many cases of broken compensation, and in cases with high blood pressure even while compensation is still good, salines administered once or twice a week assist in elimination, and in the reduction of blood pressure.

However, profuse purging in heart disease may be followed by unfavorable symptoms, especially when the systolic blood pressure is low. When there is hypotension, or when the diastolic pressure is high and the venous pressure is high, and when there is edema or effusion, watery catharsis should be caused only after due consideration, and always with a careful watching of the effect on the heart and blood pressure. The blood pressure is lowered by such catharsis, and the heart is often slowed. Neilson and Hyland [Footnote: Neilson, C. H., and Hyland, R. F.: The Effect of Strong Purging on Blood Pressure and the Heart, THE JOURNAL A. M. A., Feb. 8, 1913, p. 436.] studied the effect of purging on the heart and blood pressure, and were inclined to the view that in serious heart conditions brisk purging should not be done. They think that the slowing of the heart after such purging may be, due to an increased viscosity of the blood, or perhaps to a reflex irritation from the purgative on the intestinal canal.

Pilcher and Sollmann [Footnote: Pilcher and Sollmann: Jour. Pharmacol. and Exper. Therap., 1913, vi, 323.] have shown that the fall of blood pressure after the administration of nitrites is mostly due to the action of these drugs on the peripheral vessels. Chloroform, of course, depressed the vasomotor center, but ether had no effect on this center, or slightly stimulated it. Such stimulation, however, Pilcher and Sollmann believe may be secondary to asphyxia. Nicotin they found to cause intense stimulation of the vasomotor center. Ergot and hydrastis and its alkaloids seem to have no effect on the vasomotor center. Strophanthus acted on this center only moderately, and digitalis very slightly, if at all. Camphor in doses large enough to cause convulsions stimulated the vasomotor center. In smaller doses it generally stimulated the center moderately, but not always. Even when this center was stimulated, however, the camphor did not necessarily increase the blood pressure. The rise in blood pressure from epinephrin is due entirely to its action on the peripheral blood vessels and the heart. It has no action on the vasomotor center. They found that strychnin in large doses may stimulate the vasomotor center moderately, but usually it did not act on this center unless the patient was asphyxiated; then it acted intensely. The conclusion to be drawn from their experiments is that when there is asphyxia, increased venous pressure, and also a rising blood pressure from the stimulation of carbon dioxid, strychnin is contraindicated.

It should be recognized that digitalis very frequently not only does not raise blood pressure, but also may lower it; especially in aortic insufficiency and when there is cyanosis. Even with some forms of angina pectoris, digitalis in small doses may reduce the frequency of the pain. This decrease of pain following the use of digitalis has in some cases been ascribed to the improvement of coronary circulation and resulting better nutrition of heart muscle. Of course under these conditions the action of digitalis must be carefully watched, and it should not be given too long.

Although sodium nitrite and nitroglycerin have but a short period of action, in laboratory experimentation, in lowering the blood pressure, when given repeatedly four or five times a day the blood pressure is lowered in very many instances by these drugs. Sometimes when the blood pressure is not lowered, there is relief of tension in the head from high pressure, and the patient feels better. There is also relief of the heart when it is laboring to overcome a high resistance. One drop of the official spirit of nitroglycerin on the tongue will cause a lowering in the peripheral pressure pulse, the radial pulse becoming larger and fuller. This effect begins in three minutes or less, reaches its maximum in about five minutes, and the effect passes off in fifteen minutes or more. [Footnote: Hewlett, A. W., and Zwaluwenburg, J. G. Van: The Pulse Flow in the Brachial Artery, Arch. Int. Med., July, 1913, p. 1.]

It has been stated that iodids are of no value except in syphilitic arteriosclerosis, but iodids in small doses are stimulant to the thyroid gland, and the thyroid secretes a vasodilating substance. Therefore, the use of either iodids or thyroid would seem to be justified in many instances of high blood pressure.

Fairlee [Footnote: Fairlee: Lancet, London, Feb. 28, 1914.] has studied the effect of chloroform and ether on blood pressure, and finds that there is a fall of pressure throughout the administration of chloroform, and but little alteration of the blood pressure during the administration of ether. It may cause a slight rise, or it may cause a slight fall, but changes in pressure with ether are not marked. When there is slight surgical shock present, as from some injury, they found that chloroform would lower the pressure considerably. Hence it would seem that chloroform should not be used as an anesthetic after serious injuries.

THE EFFECT OF DRUGS ON VENOUS BLOOD PRESSURE

Capps and Matthews [Footnote: Capps, J. A., and Matthews, S. A.: Venous Blood Pressure as influenced by the Drugs Employed in Cardiovascular Therapy, THE JOURNAL A. M. A., Aug. 9, 1913, p. 388.] have shown that even with first class preparations of digitalis, there may be only a moderate gradual rise in arterial pressure, but not much change in venous pressure. Venous pressure was not much affected by small doses of epinephrin, but with large doses it rose from 10 to 80 mm. Pituitary extract acts somewhat similarly to epinephrin. Caffein, though raising the arterial pressure, did not influence the venous pressure. Strychnin did not raise either pressure until the dose was sufficient to cause muscular contractions. They found that the nitrites caused a fall in venous pressure as well as arterial pressure, although the heart might be accelerated and more regular. They think that the nitrites act by depressing the nerve endings in the veins as well as the arteries. Morphin they found did not act on the venous pressure, although it lowered arterial tension, in ordinary doses of 1/8 or 1/6 grain; but with doses of from 1/4 to 1/2 grain, both arterial and venous pressures were lowered. They found that alcohol in ordinary doses did not influence the venous pressure, although it lowered the arterial pressure; but very large doses lowered the arterial and raised the venous pressure. They think that when the venous pressure is increased only by large doses of epinephrin, pituitary extract and alcohol, the effect is due to failure of the heart, although it may be due to an increase of carbon dioxid in the blood, in other words, to asphyxia.

HYPERTENSION

Arterial hypertension may be divided into stages. In the first stage the arteries are healthy, but the tone, owing to contraction of the muscular walls, is too great. This condition or stage has been termed "chronic arterial hypertension." This condition may be due to irritants circulating in the blood, to nervous tension, to incipient chronic interstitial nephritis, or may be the first stage of sclerosis of the arteries. If from any cause this hypertension persists, the muscular coats of the arteries will become more or less hypertrophied, and sooner or later degenerative changes begin in the intima, and finally fibrosis occurs in the external coat of the arteries; in other words, arteriosclerosis is in evidence. If the patient lives with this arteriosclerosis, a later stage of the arterial disease may occur which has been termed atheroma, with thickening, and possibly calcareous deposits in some parts of the walls of the vessels, while in other parts the coats become thinner and insufficient. At this stage the heart, which has already shown some trouble, becomes unable to force the blood properly against this enormous resistance of inelastic vessels and the blood pressure begins to fail as the left ventricle weakens.

Edema, failing heart, perhaps aneurysms, peripheral obstruction, or hemorrhages are the final conditions in this chronic disease of arteriosclerosis.

Riesman [Footnote: Riesman: Pennsylvania Med. Jour., December, 1911, p. 193.] divides hypertension into four classes hypertension without apparent nephritis or arterial disease; hypertension with arteriosclerosis; hypertension with nephritis, and hypertension with both arteriosclerosis and nephritis. These classes are given here in the order of the seriousness of the prognosis.

ETIOLOGY

One of the most common causes of hypertension is clue to excess of eating and drinking. The products caused by maldigestion of proteins, and the toxins formed and absorbed especially from meat proteins, particularly when the excretions are insufficient, are the most frequent causes of hypertension. Whatever other element or condition may have caused increased blood pressure, the first step toward improving and lowering this pressure is to diminish the amount of meat eaten or to remove it entirely from the diet. In pregnancy where there is increased metabolic change, when the proteins are not well or properly cared for in gout, and when there is intestinal fermentation or putrefaction, hypertension is likely to occur. The increased blood pressure in these cases is directly due to irritation of the toxins on the blood vessel walls.

While alcohol does not tend to raise arterial blood pressure, in large amounts it may raise the venous pressure. Also, by causing an abundant appetite and thus increasing the amount of food taken, by interfering with the activity of the liver, and by impairing the intestinal digestion, it can indirectly disturb the metabolism and cause enough toxin to be produced to raise the blood pressure.

Any drug or substance that raises the blood pressure by stimulating the vasomotor center or the arterioles, when constantly repeated, will be a cause of hypertension. This is particularly true of caffein and nicotin. Also, anything that might stimulate, or that does stimulate, the suprarenal glands will cause a continued high blood pressure. It is quite probable that in many cases of gout the suprarenals are hypersecreting and it has been shown by Cannon, Aub and Binger [Footnote: Cannon, Aub and Binger: Jour. Pharmacol. and Exper. Therap., March, 1912.] that nicotin in small closes increases the suprarenal secretion. Therefore, nicotin becomes a decided cause of hypertension and arteriosclerosis.

Thayer found that heavy work is the cause of about two thirds of all cases of arteriosclerosis, and one of the functions of the suprarenals is to destroy the waste products of muscular activity; hence these glands, in these cases, are hypersecreting. Furthermore, the reason that many infections are followed later by arterio- sclerosis may be the fact that the suprarenals have been stimulated to hypertrophy and hypersecrete.

Many persons in middle life, and especially women at the time of the menopause, show hypertension without arterial or kidney reason. At this time of life the thyroid is disturbed, and often, especially if weight is added, it is not secreting sufficiently. Whether, with the polyglandular disturbance of the menopause the suprarenals are excited and hypersecreting, or whether they are simply relatively secreting more vasopressor substance than is combated by the vasodilator substance from the thyroid, cannot be determined. These women are energetic, and look full of health and full of strength, but their faces frequently flush, sometimes they are dizzy, and the systolic blood pressure is too high. Reisman has pointed out that these patients are likely to have very large breasts, and there is reason to believe that we must begin to study more carefully the effect of large breasts on the metabolism of girls and women. There certainly is an internal secretion of some importance furnished by these glands.

In hyperthyroidism at first the blood pressure may be lowered on account of the increased physiologic secretion of the thyroid gland. Later the blood pressure may be raised by stimulation of the suprarenals, or it may become raised from the irritated and stimulated heart becoming hypertrophied. If the heart is normal the ventricles should hypertrophy with the increased work that they are under; and the blood pressure could increase for this reason. Later in exophthalmic goiter the heart muscle may become degenerated, a chronic myocarditis, and the ventricles may slightly dilate. At this time the blood pressure is lowered. When such a condition has occurred, the heart bears thyroidectomy badly; hence an operation on this gland should, if possible, be performed before the heart muscle has become injured. If the heart shows signs of loss of power, minor operations to cut off the blood supply of the thyroid should first be done, and the patient's heart allowed to improve before a thyroidectomy is performed.

Men with hypertension without kidney or arterial excuse are likely to have been athletes, or to have done some severe competitive work, or, as above stated, to have labored hard, or to have worked at high tension, or in great excitement, or with mental worry, all of which tend, as long as there is health, to increase the blood pressure. These men may add weight from the age of 40 on, or they may be thin and wiry. Besides the hypertension there is likely to be a too sturdily acting heart, which is often hypertrophied, and there is an accentuated closure of the aortic valve. There may be dizziness, or no head symptoms at all. Nicotin is likely to be an etiologic factor in this class.

These women and these men may all be improved by proper treatment, and the condition may not develop into arteriosclerosis or nephritis.

Neurotic conditions, and in some instances neurasthenic conditions, may show a blood pressure higher than normal. Lead may be a cause of increased blood pressure, and diabetics occasionally have a high pressure, although more frequently there is a lowering of blood pressure in diabetes.

Richman believes that syphilis is the most common cause of hypertension and arteriosclerosis without renal disease. When arteriosclerosis and renal disease are combined, of course the highest systolic readings occur. He thinks that when high tension occurs under 40 years of age, kidney disease is generally the cause. Of course it may be the only cause later in life.

High blood pressure due to syphilitic conditions may be greatly improved by the proper treatment, although some one or more blood vessels are likely to have been seriously damaged. Although these patients may live for many years, they are likely to have an apoplexy, cerebral disease or an aneurysm.

While hypertension is not a disease, and while it often should not be combated, still, as it is always the forerunner of more serious trouble, there can be no excuse for not most seriously considering it and generally attempting its reduction. At the moment high tension is discovered, there may be no special symptoms; but troublesome symptoms are always pending, and while the patient need not be unduly alarmed, there is no excuse for not rearranging the individual's life so as to prolong it. This is not to state that every high tension must be lowered, but every hypertension must be studied and a safer systolic pressure caused if it is possible without interfering with the person's efficiency. A high diastolic pressure, one above 105, certainly must receive immediate attention, and a diastolic pressure of 110 must be lowered, if possible. On the other hand, a high systolic pressure without a high diastolic pressure should not be rapidly lowered, else depression will be caused.

SYMPTOMS

In hypertension, as long as the heart, which is probably hypertrophied, remains perfectly competent, there are few symptoms, and the person does not seek advice until he notices one or more of several possible conditions. He may be dizzy, his head may feel full and tight, he may have headaches, or he may have some cardiac pain or distress. Other persons do not seek advice until there is a slight weakening of the heart, showing the strain under which it is laboring. In most of these high tension cases, the patients have rather a slow heart, provided the heart is sufficient. Eyster and Hooker [Footnote: Eyster and Hooker: Am. Jour. Physiol., May, 1908.] found that the slowing of the heart in high blood pressure is due to action through the vagus nerves either from the inhibitory center in the medulla or reflexly by stimulation of the peripheral nerves of the vessels.

Another symptom for which the patient frequently seeks advice is that he is unable to relax from his business cares, when off duty. He also finds that he works at a higher tension, and that coffee and tea, alcohol and tobacco stimulate him more than usual. He sleeps restlessly, and dreams at night. He has an increased frequency of urination in the morning, especially after taking coffee, and sometimes gets up once or twice at night to urinate. He is irritable at times; short breathed on exertion, and sometimes has indigestion. He may have pains or aches in his heart. He may find that he dislikes to lie on his left side.

However much it may upset the patient and render him more nervous to inform him that his blood pressure is too high, it is necessary to give him this information. People now suspect the condition, and they frequently seek their physicians to determine if the blood pressure is too high and, from reading health journals, more or less realize some of the things, at least, that must be done to decrease the pressure. Consequently, the very things that are advised or ordered give the patient the diagnosis, whether he is told directly or not. Hence, we must talk freely with the patient, much as we do in heart defects, and get his cooperation, stating how frequent the condition is, how often it is readily improved, and how little it may interfere with long life.

Wiener and Wolfner [Footnote: Wiener, Meyer, and Wolfner, M. L.: A Reaction of the Pupil, Strongly Suggestive of Arteriosclerosis with Increased Blood Pressure, THE JOURNAL A. M. A., July 17, 1915, p. 214.] state that they have found with blood pressure that the pupils of the eyes are larger than normal, and that they readily contract to the stimulus of light, but immediately return to their previous size.

PROGNOSIS

Janeway [Footnote: Janeway, T. C.: A Clinical Study of Hypertensive Cardiovascular Disease, Arch. Int. Med., December, 1913, p. 755.] presented statistics of 458 patients with high blood pressure, 67 percent of whom were men. Of these 458 patients 212 had died, and he found that the women with high blood pressure lived longer than men with high blood pressure. They did not seem as likely to have apoplexy or cardiac failure. About 85 percent of high tension cases occur between the ages of 40 and 70.

While he believes that a systolic pressure of over 160 mm. is pathologic, he does not find that any definite prognostic conclusions can be drawn from the height of the pressure. Of course the most important concomitant symptoms of high pressure are cardiac, renal, and cerebral, and the typical headache, as he terms it, is a symptom of serious import. In considering headache in persons over 40, we must eliminate the eye headaches produced by the need of presbyopic glasses or by the need of stronger lenses, as this need is a frequent cause of headache. Dizziness and vertigo may occur without headache, and drowsiness, though not so frequent a symptom as insomnia, often occurs.

Janeway finds that all kinds of apoplectic attacks may occur from simple transient aphasia to complete hemiplegia, and thirteen of his patients who had died and thirteen of those living at the time of this report showed failure of eyesight as an initial symptom of arterial disease.

Janeway deplores the too frequent diagnosis of neurasthenia in these patients. This diagnosis probably accounts for the frequency with which neurasthenics have been said to have high blood pressure. Patients with high blood pressure may show all kinds of symptoms simulating neurasthenia, but hypertension is a much better diagnosis than neurasthenia for such patients, and will lead to more rational treatment.

Ninety-seven of these patients had hemorrhages somewhere, most frequently epistaxes, sometimes hemoptysis. Janeway did not find that purpuric spots on the skin occurred early in the disease in any of his patients.

Gastro-intestinal disturbances were not much in evidence unless the kidneys were insufficient. Intermittent claudication in the legs occasionally occurred. While angina pectoris and edema of the lungs were not infrequent causes of death in men, it was a rare cause of death in women. Dyspnea is a frequent symptom, and one for which many patients seek medical advice.

A constant systolic blood pressure of over 200 shows a probability that the patient will ultimately die either of uremia or of apoplexy. Janeway found that those patients who are to die from cardiac weakness show cardiac symptoms early in their disease. He found that rapid continuous loss of weight pointed to an early fatal termination.

Of the 212 patients who had died, seventy-one had shown cardiac insufficiency at the time of the first examination; twenty-one showed albumin or casts at that time. Of course it should be repeatedly emphasized that chronic interstitial nephritis may be in evidence with either albumin or casts alone, or without either being present.

Janeway sums up his conclusions by stating that "from the time of the development of symptoms indicative of cardiovascular or renal disease, four years will witness the death of half the men and five years of half the women. By the tenth year half the remainder will have died, leaving one fourth both of the men and the women who have lived beyond ten years." The causes of death he would place in the following order: gradual cardiac failure; uremia; apoplexy; some complicating acute infection; angina pectoris; accidental causes; acute edema of the lungs and cachexia. An early occurrence of myocardial weakness shows a 50 percent probability that death will be caused by cardiac insufficiency. Heart pains comprise another important indicator of future cardiac death, perhaps not an angina. Nocturnal polyuria would indicate a uremic death in about 50 percent of the patients, and typical headache or cerebral symptoms show the probability of uremic death in more than 50 percent, and death from apoplexy in a large number of the other 50 percent As just stated, rapid loss of weight is a bad symptom.

Janeway [Footnote: Janeway, T. C.: A Study of the Causes of Death in One Hundred Patients with High Blood Pressure, THE JOURNAL A. M. A., Dec. 14, 1912, p. 2106.] has previously reported seven patients with hypertension who had diabetes. Diabetes generally, on the other hand, causes a low blood pressure. Patients with this trouble and with hypertension, and without nephritis, probably have an increased secretion from the suprarenals.

We may sum up the prognosis in hypertension as follows: Hypertension alone is not of unfavorable omen; if it is not readily reduced by ordinary means, it is more serious. If associated with kidney, heart or liver defect, it is most serious. If there are such serious conditions as edema, ascites, lung congestion, cyanosis and great dyspnea, the prognosis is dire.

Obesity being a cause of high blood pressure, it should be treated more or less energetically, even if the individual does not continue to add weight.

Stone [Footnote: Stone, W. J.: The Differentiation of Cerebral and Cardiac Types of Hyperarterial Tension in Vascular Disease, Arch. Int. Med., November, 1915, p. 775.] believes that the higher the diastolic pressure the greater danger there is of cerebral death, while a patient with a very high systolic, but a diastolic pressure of 100 or lower, is in more danger of cardiac death. He urges a greater consideration of the pressure pulse in determining the load of the heart and the great danger from a sustained diastolic pressure of over 105 as sooner or later bound to cause myocardial symptoms. This load of the heart is also shown by an increased pulse rate and increased respiratory efforts. In cardiac failure, as the systolic pressure falls the diastolic is likely to be increased, and the pressure pulse thus diminishing, allows insufficient blood to go to the medullary centers, and death soon occurs. Therefore, in acute illnesses a sustained pressure pulse gives a better prognosis than a diminishing pressure pulse. The strenuous measures that should he used to lower a high diastolic pressure are contraindicated when the diastolic pressure is already low, even if the systolic pressure 1s high. If a high systolic pressure begins to fall more or less rapidly the heart shows fatigue, and should be stimulated by digitalis or strophanthin.

Rowan [Footnote: Rowan, J. J.: The Practical Application of Blood Pressure Findings, THE JOURNAL A. M. A., March 18, 1916, p. 873.] finds that a diastolic reading of 100 mm. or more usually means that there is a narrowing of the lumen of the vessels, owing to stimulation of the vasoconstrictors, although it may mean the existence of a true arterial fibrosis. While a real atheroma generally causes a reduction in diastolic blood pressure, or at least but slight increase, he has found in syphilitic cases with arteriosclerosis a high diastolic pressure. If the blood pressure cannot be reduced by ordinary measures, arteriosclerosis is probably present. Several blood pressure examinations must be made, while the patient is being treated, to establish the diagnosis.

Rowan finds the reading of the pulse pressure to be of great importance, as this will indicate, sometimes before any other symptom is present, that the patient is either improving or doing badly, and it also aids in indicating the proper medicinal treatment.

In arteriosclerosis the systolic pressure may be high while the diastolic is low; hence there is a large pressure pulse. If the heart becomes weak the systolic pressure will drop, and any improvement caused, especially in aortic regurgitation, is by an increase of the systolic pressure.

Rowan finds, as has long been recognized, that a conclusion as to whether or not cerebral hemorrhage will occur cannot be made from the condition of the radial arteries, as patients with soft radials may suffer from cerebral hemorrhage, while those "with hard, sclerosed, pipestem-like arteries may live to a great age and die of anything rather than apoplexy."

Swan, [Footnote: Swan: Interstate Med. Jour., March, 1915, p. 186.] has studied the blood pressure in fifty cases of disturbed thyroid, and finds that functional myocardial tests show that the myocardium is nearly always disturbed in these patients.

Before taking up the subject of treatment of high blood pressure, it may be suggested that a high diastolic pressure with a falling systolic pressure may require vasodilators on the one hand or cardiac tonics on the other, and sometimes the decision can be made only by proper tests. In other words, if the diastolic pressure is lowered the heart will be relieved. On the other hand, if the diastolic is being raised by an increased venous pressure from a failing heart, digitalis, strychnin and caffein may be of benefit in lowering the diastolic as well as raising the systolic. However, if there is a high systolic and a low diastolic pressure, vasodilators are often contraindicated.

TREATMENT

In this rapid high tension age the physician should be as energetic in teaching prevention of arterial hypertension as he is in preventing contagion. As infectious diseases are reduced in frequency, more patients live to die of diseases later in life, and (as previously stated) diseases with hypertension are on the increase. It is therefore the duty of the physician to urge youths and adults to abstain from all kinds of excesses so common in this age. We live at such speed, even the children, that this caution is almost daily needed. We must caution against severe athletic competition, against personal "stunts," against recreation excesses, even golfing, automobiling and dancing, against excess in the use of tobacco, in eating, in late dinners, in coffee, tea and alcohol. We must take better care of patients during their convalescence from some serious illness lest they have circulatory debility by becoming strenuous too soon after their recovery. The pregnant woman must be more carefully watched, not only for her own sake, but also for the sake of her child. Intestinal indigestion, while not the cause of all disturbances that occur in man after 40, is still an important element in his deterioration and degeneration, and it should be prevented if possible.

The tendency for hypertension and arteriosclerosis to occur early in life in patients who have suffered some serious acute infection, whether blood poisoning, typhoid fever, or other, shows that in all probability in these acute illnesses the internal secretions are so disturbed that the suprarenal activity is greater than normal, while the thyroid activity may be less than normal, and hypertension is the consequence. Therefore, these infected patients who recover should probably have a longer convalescence in order for the more delicate structures of the body, such as the internal secreting glands, to have a better chance to recover and become normal.

The enumeration of these causes and the causes that have been mentioned before not only suggest, but also direct the treatment of hypertension after it has occurred. The most important of all treatment for hypertension is rest. That means for an individual, well except for his hypertension, a vacation, that is, a rest from physical and mental labor. For a patient who is in serious trouble from hypertension, bed rest is the most important element in the management. As has been previously shown, good sleep lowers the blood pressure, and Brooks and Carroll [Footnote: Brooks, Harlow, and Carroll, J. H.; A Clinical Study of the Effects of Sleep and Rest on Blood Pressure, Arch. Int. Med., August, 1912, p. 97.] showed that the greatest drop in blood pressure occurs in the first part of the night's sleep. In other words, a patient who lies awake long loses the best part of his night's rest as far as his circulation is concerned. This is one more reason for abstinence from tea and coffee in the evening by those patients who are at all disturbed by the caffein. On the other hand, patients who are not seriously ill should not remain for days in bed, as the blood pressure does not tend to continue to fall, although the heart may become weakened by such bed rest. This is especially true if the patient is nervous and irritable and objects to such confinement.

A systolic pressure much over 200 probably never goes down to normal, and if such a high systolic pressure goes down to below 170, we should consider the treatment successful.

Every active treatment of hypertension should begin with a thorough cleaning out of the intestinal canal by purgation, best with mercury in some form. Then the diet should be modified to meet the individual case and the person's activity. If the blood pressure is dangerously high, he should receive but little nourishment, best in the form of cereals and skimmed milk.

On the other hand, if he has edema or dropsy, or if the heart showed signs of weakness, large amounts of liquids should certainly not be given, and in such cases it is better that he receive small quantities of milk if that agrees, rather than large quantities of skimmed milk. The amount of water should also be fitted to the circulatory ability and the condition of the kidneys.

When more or less active treatment does not soon lower the hypertension, and especially a high diastolic pressure, the prognosis is bad. In a patient who is in more or less immediate danger from his hypertension, the food and liquid taken, the care of the bowels, and the measures used to cause secretions from the skin must all be governed by the condition of his other organs. There is no excuse for excessive, strenuous measures when the heart is failing or when the kidneys are becoming progressively insufficient. Strenuosity in treatment is as objectionable in these cases as is neglect of treatment in earlier stages of the trouble.

Bie [Footnote: Bie: Ugesk. f. Laeger, March 4, 1915.] believes there is no direct connection between the blood pressure and the anatomic condition in the kidneys, although abnormal conditions in the two are almost invariably found parallel.

A patient with simple hypertension and otherwise well, which means that his diastolic pressure is at least no higher than 110, should have his diet, tobacco, coffee and tea regulated; should have recreation periods one or more times a week, and vacations not too infrequently; should take some brisk purgative once or twice a week, and may receive one or other of the physical treatments for the reduction of blood pressure, whether Turkish baths or electric light baths. If he does not sleep well, there is no hypnotic drug so valuable in his case as chloral. This should not be long given, but it will produce the purest kind of sleep and lowers the blood pressure.

If any other drug is needed, nitroglycerin is the best. If arteriosclerosis is present, sodium iodid in small doses, 3 grains two or three times a day, is valuable. Larger doses of sodium iodid are not needed, unless it is advisable to give such doses for a short period. The value of iodid in these cases is best obtained by small doses long continued. If the patient is obese, shall doses of thyroid extract long continued are of value, such as 2 or 3 grains once a day. If the thyroid extract causes the heart to become more rapid, it should be discontinued.

Whether the diet should be meat protein free, or whether meat may be allowed once a day, depends entirely on the individual and on his physical activities. It is frequently a mistake to take all meat out of his diet.

When there is obesity, the bulk of the food should be greatly diminished, and anything that tends to stimulate the patient's appetite should be withheld. This means all condiments, and at times even salt. Sugar should be greatly reduced, and starches greatly reduced, but he must have some. In other words, he should not be cut down to a diabetic diet. No more liquid should be taken with the meals than is essential to swallow the food. Water should be taken between meals. There is no question that almost every one today should have a very light breakfast, except perhaps those who labor hard physically and are exposed for hours, daily, to the inclemencies of the weather. Such patients probably need more food. It is also well, in hypertension cases, to have one day a week in which a very minimum amount of food is taken, whether that be milk, or skimmed milk, or a small amount of carbohydrate, without protein food.

If the foregoing management does not reduce hypertension, the kidneys are generally beginning to become involved in the sclerotic degeneration, whether the urine shows such a condition or not. On the other hand, there are exceptions to this rule.

As indican in the urine gives evidence of putrefactive changes in the intestines and the probability of the absorption of toxins from the intestines, although we have no real proof that these toxins are the direct cause of hypertension, our patient is undoubtedly physically better, and will have less arterial tension when this intestinal condition is removed. Therefore, our treatment of the individual is not a success as long as such fermentation and putrefaction persist. If such putrefaction cannot be removed by diet and laxatives and mental rest and the prevention of physical strenuosity, radical changes in diet are advisable, although it may not be necessary to continue such a diet more than a few days at a time. A rigid milk diet for a few days may change the flora of the intestine completely; then a vegetable diet may be given, with return to a mixed diet; or the various lactic acid bacilli may be given, or one of the various fermented milks may be the diet, the object being to change the flora in the intestine and thus modify the ferments. So-called bowel antiseptics, such as salol, for a short time may be of advantage. Colon washings may be of great advantage. Liquid petroleum may be advantageous.

Besides preventing the absorption of toxins from the intestine, we must prevent such absorption from any latent infection. The most frequent kind of such infection is pyorrhea alveolaris.

A simple method that sometimes is an efficient aid in lowering the blood pressure is complete muscular and mental relaxation. The patient lies down for a while in the middle of the day and relaxes every muscle of his body. With this he may take slow breathing exercises. He should be in a dark room, quiet if possible, and alone, and should teach his brain to be for a short time mentally inert.

The physical methods of lowering the blood pressure are hydrotherapeutic, whether by warm baths or more strenuously by Turkish baths, by hot air baths (body baking) which is occasionally very efficient, or, perhaps more now in vogue, by electric light baths. The duration of these baths, and the frequency, must be determined by the results. If the heart is made rapid, and the heart muscle shows signs of weakness, the duration of these baths must not be long, and they may be contraindicated. These baths are most efficient in lowering the blood pressure when the patient reclines for several hours after the bath. The amount of sweating that is advisable in these cases depends on the condition of the heart. If the heart muscle is insufficient, profuse sweating is inadvisable. Also if the kidneys are insufficient, profuse sweating is inadvisable as tending to concentrate the toxins in the blood. On the other hand, when the surface of the body tends to be cool, and there are internal congestions, the value of these baths is very great. Sometimes the electric light baths increase the tension instead of diminishing it, and when properly used they may be of benefit in some cases of hypotension. The frequency of the baths and the question of how many weeks they should be intermittently continued, depend on the individual case. After a course of such treatment sometimes patients have a diminished systolic blood pressure not only for weeks, but even for months, provided they do not break the rules laid down for them.

The Nauheim baths, while stated not to raise the blood pressure, are not much advocated in hypertension, and Brown [Footnote: Brown: California State Jour. Med., November, 1907, p. 279.] who made more than 500 observations of patients of all ages, found that the full strength Nauheim bath would raise the blood pressure in all feverish and circulatory conditions. He also found that a fifteen minute sodium chlorid bath, 7 pounds to 40 gallons, at a temperature of from 94 to 98 degrees F., lowered the pressure from 10 to 15 mm. This is not different from the effect obtained from a fifteen minute warm bath at from 94 to 98 degrees F., or a fifteen minute mustard bath of the same temperature. In other words, the slight irritation of mustard or of salt in a warm bath made no special difference in the amount of lowering of the blood pressure. On the other hand, he found that a fifteen minute calcium chlorid bath, 1 1/2 pounds to 40 gallons, at 94 degrees F., raised the blood pressure 15 mm.

The autocondensation treatment to lower the blood pressure is not so satisfactory as it was hoped to be. The blood pressure can thus be lowered, but it soon again rises, and probably generally more rapidly than after the bath treatments, and in some persons it causes considerable depression. Van Rennselaer [Footnote: Van Rensselaer: Month. Cycl. and Med. Bull., November, 1912, p. 643.] has reviewed this subject of high frequency treatment, and recalls the fact that Nicola Tesla demonstrated, in 1891, the form of electricity which we now term high frequency. High frequency means more than 10,000 cycles per second, at which frequency muscles do not contract and pain is not felt, whereas in medicine the frequency of the currents used runs up into the hundreds of thousands, or even into the millions. The French investigator, d'Arsonval, studied the physiologic action of these high frequency currents and found that the respiration and heart are made more rapid and the blood pressure is reduced, while the intake of oxygen is increased and the carbon dioxid excretion is increased. The temperature may rise. The excretion of the urinary solids is mostly increased. Perspiration may be caused, and he believes the glandular activities are increased. In a word, metabolic changes in the body are made more active and the blood pressure is lowered.

Besides the effect of altitude on blood pressure, as previously declared, patients with dangerously high blood pressure should, if possible, not be subjected to intense cold. In other words, a person with hyper-tension, if financially able, should not remain in a cold climate during the winter. On the other hand, even if he is stout and feels sufficiently warm with light clothing during the winter, his skin becoming chilled adds to his tension. Therefore he should be clothed as warmly as he will tolerate.

After a period which may be termed the normal period of hypertension in normal life, as age advances the systolic tension may lower, provided there is no kidney lesion. This is due to the slowly developing chronic myocarditis and a lessening of the tension and therefore lessening of the resistance to the heart. This may be nature's method of lengthening the life of the individual. In other words, as the arteries grow older the force of the heart slightly lessens, the blood pressure lowers, and the individual is safer. This frequently occurs in otherwise perfectly normal individuals, without treatment.

When the blood pressure is suddenly excessively high from any cause, venesection may be life saving, and should perhaps be more frequently done than it is. It may save a heart that is in agony from tension, and may prevent an apoplexy. It is of little value except temporarily in uremic conditions, but at other times it may, at the time, save life and allow other methods of reducing the dangerous tension to become effective. A chronic high tension patient may be repeatedly bled, although such treatment will not long save life, as the blood pressure in many such cases soon returns to its previous height.

Some very high tension cases, especially in women at the menopause, and where there is no kidney involvement, have the blood pressure reduced successfully only by large doses of thyroid, sometimes well combined with bromids, especially if the thyroid causes excitation. Such treatment persisted in for a time may cause months of improvement, and even years.

DRUGS IN HYPERTENSION

The drugs that are mostly used to lower blood pressure are nitrites or drugs which are like nitrites, and these are nitroglycerin, sodium nitrite, erythroltetra nitrate and amyl nitrite, and the frequency of their use is in the order named. Other drugs used to lower blood pressure are iodids, thyroid, alkalies, chloral, bromids and aconite, the latter rarely.

Amyl nitrite is required only when a sudden immediate effect is desired in angina pectoris or in some other serious spasmodic condition. Sodium nitrite is more likely to upset the stomach than is nitroglycerin. It acts, however, a little longer, but not enough to warrant its frequent selection. The dose of sodium nitrite is from 0.03 to 0.06 gm. (1/2 grain to a grain), best in tablet form and given with plenty of water. The tablet should of course be dissolved or crushed with the teeth. It should not be given on an empty stomach, as it may cause considerable irritation and pain. It more or less actively lowers the blood pressure for about an hour.

Erythrol tetranitrate is preferred by some clinicians who find that its effect lasts somewhat longer. There is probably, however, no better nitrite or nitrate than nitroglycerin. While it acts but a short time, it acts effectively, and although no nitrite has vasodilating effects for any length of time from one dose, when the doses are given repeatedly and for days at a time, the blood pressure will generally be more or less reduced. The dose is from 1/500 to 1/100 grain, three or four times a day, or every three hours, as desired. The best form in which to use it is in a very soluble tablet, and the tablet should not be dissolved unless intense immediate action is desired. It acts when absorbed from the tongue almost as rapidly as when given hypodermically; it acts in two or three minutes, and the blood pressure may drop from 20 to 30 mm. In experimental tests the action does not last more than from fifteen minutes to half an hour, but clinically the effect of repeated doses is much more satisfactory. Spirit of glyceryl trinitrate or spirit of Nitroglycerin, dose 1 minim, keeps well if care is taken to guard against evaporation of alcohol; tablets if well made and kept in bottles properly corked, will retain their activity for months.

The closer a physician is to the laboratory, the less he believes in the value of nitroglycerin in hypertension. The nearer he is to clinical work the more he believes in it. It is a fact that in some instances, even with a dose as small as 1/200 grain of nitroglycerin, three or four times in twenty-four hours, the blood pressure will be lower, whatever the diet is and whatever the other treatments are, than if the patient does not take the nitroglycerin. Also the value of these short relaxation periods from the standpoint of a strained and tired heart should not be underestimated, the same as the value of a night's rest, or the value of a recreation period of an hour or two. If a patient has hypotension and a systolic pressure of 110, and is given nitroglycerin, the very unpleasant results from its administration will be immediately noticed. Hence nitroglycerin is one of the most valuable drugs that we possess for the treatment of hypertension, and some patients are even benefited by as small a dose as l/500 grain. Lawrence [Footnote: Lawrence, C. H.: The Effect of Pressure-Lowering Drugs and Therapeutic Measures on Systolic and Diastolic Pressure in Man, Arch. Int. Med., April, 1912, p. 409.] found that the fall of diastolic pressure from nitrites was about half of the fall of systolic pressure. When there is no kidney lesion a very high systolic pressure falls more under nitroglycerin than does a medium high systolic pressure.

Alkalies, whether potassium or sodium citrate or sodium bicarbonate, are often of advantage in so changing and aiding metabolism, or perhaps reducing the irritation from hyperacidity or a mild condition of acidosis, that their administration causes a lowering of blood pressure.

While iodids may not be direct vasodilators and do not render the blood more aplastic or diminish its viscosity, as shown by Capps [Footnote: Capps, J. A.: Effect of Iodids on the Circulation and Blood

Vessels in Arteriosclerosis, THE JOURNAL A. M. A., Oct. 12, 1912. p. 1350.] still, iodids in small doses, 0.1 to 0.2 gm. (1-1/2 to 3 grains) given from once to three times a day, after meals (these small doses do not disturb the stomach), will stimulate the thyroid gland to greater activity, and when this gland secretes properly, the blood pressure is somewhat lowered. Of course, in syphilitic sclerosis large doses of iodids are indicated and are valuable.

In obese patients with hypertension, in the hypertension of women at the menopause, and in hypertension with insufficient kidneys, thyroid medication is often of great value. Sometimes a small dose of from 0.1 to 0.2 gm. (1 1/12 to 3 grains) once a day is all that is needed. At other times, especially when there is no marked arteriosclerosis and no marked kidney or liver lesion, very high blood pressures are reduced only by very large doses, even as much as 10 grains a day. Such treatment is often of very great benefit. Of course, if one of the persons under consideration has symptoms of hyperthyroidism, or if small doses of thyroid cause palpitation, the treatment is not indicated, on the one hand, and should be stopped, on the other. Sometimes when the blood pressure cannot be reduced, in these cases without apparent organic lesions, and thyroid treatment is more or less successful, but at the same time causes great excitation, it may be combined with bromid medication, and then the benefit is sometimes very great.

A patient who cannot sleep and who has hypertension may receive bromids if he is very irritable or if there are symptoms of thyroid irritability; but the most successful sleep and lowering of blood pressure is caused by chloral. A dose of 0.5 gm. (7 1/2 grains) at night is generally sufficient and need not be long continued. Chloral has been frequently given to reduce pressure in 0.2 to 0.25 gm. (3 or 4 grain) doses, three times a day, after meals.

Bromids, of course, will lower the blood pressure, but they depress all metabolism, interfere with digestion, and are not advisable for any length of time. However, in some cases they cause a marked improvement in the patient's condition.

Patients under treatment with chloral, bromids, and thyroid especially, should be carefully watched and the treatment modified to meet the varying conditions. Patients under iodid need not be seen so frequently; those under nitroglycerin or alkalies still less frequently. But all patients under the active management of hypertension should be seen at from one to three week intervals, and the urine should be repeatedly examined and the blood pressure carefully recorded.

HYPOTENSION

A low systolic pressure and a low diastolic pressure may not cause any symptoms or give any cause for anxiety. It does show, especially if the systolic pressure is below normal for the age of the person, a lack of reserve power, and such patients will not well stand serious illnesses, operations, injuries or serious physical and mental strains. If there is a low systolic pressure and a high diastolic pressure, this shows impairment of the heart, whether or not any other organic lesion is present.

Generally speaking, a low systolic pressure shows a weak acting heart muscle, and a very low diastolic pressure shows a dilated condition of the arterioles. In aortic regurgitation this low diastolic pressure is constantly in evidence, and, if the systolic pressure is not below normal, does not signify that the circulation is insufficient. If the systolic pressure is not very low but the diastolic is high, vasodilator drugs, by lowering the diastolic and increasing the pulse pressure, are often of benefit. If there is increased venous congestion and increased venous pressure and a high diastolic pressure with a low systolic pressure, digitalis not only will often raise the systolic pressure, but also will lower diastolic by improving the general circulation and removing venous congestion.

While intestinal indigestion and absorption of toxins often tend to raise the blood pressure, some toxins thus absorbed, especially of the ptomain variety, lower blood pressure and cause shock, perhaps by weakening the muscle of the heart or by acting on the vasodilator vessels; or they may cause dilation of the vessels of the abdomen and in this manner lower blood pressure.

Very low blood pressure after exertion, after severe physical exercise, or after competitive athletic tests shows that the heart cannot sustain such strains and should not be again subjected to them. In severe mental and physical strains the suprarenals may be inhibited in their activities, and a hypotension, more or less prolonged, may result.

Sewall [Footnote: Sewall: Am. Jour. Med. Sc., April, 1916, p. 491] believes that hypotension is frequently due to splanchnic stasis, and that sluggish circulation in this region, especially when the person is in the erect posture, is an important factor in general physiologic disturbances or lack of general tone. When the splanchnic vessels are dilated there is also a lack of proper tone to the cerebral vessels, and this may be a cause of mental weariness and neurasthenia. While ptosis of organs in the abdomen and a flaccid condition of the musculature of the abdomen are frequent causes of this splanchlnic stasis, and therefore hypotension, especially in women, it is quite possible that suprarenal insufficiency will allow this condition of the splanchnic vessels to occur frequently.

Serious illness and infections will lower the blood pressure sometimes to a dangerous point. Of course, hemorrhages lower the blood pressure. Shock and collapse cause lowering of blood pressure, frequently to a fatal point, and Cornwall [Footnote: Cornwall: New York Med. Jour. March 7, 1914, p. 470.] finds that a patient may live several hours with a systolic pressure below 60, and several days when it is below 70; that he may walk around with a systolic pressure of 90, provided the pressure pulse is sufficiently large, that is, that the diastolic pressure is low enough to cause a circulation of blood. Of course, if the difference between the systolic and the diastolic pressure is diminished to the vanishing point, the patient cannot stand it, and dies. It should be remembered that just before death venous pressure is likely to rise, and this may raise the diastolic pressure.

With the progressive toxemia of typhoid fever the blood pressure will become lowered from the myocardial degeneration. Of course, the blood pressure will drop suddenly from a hemorrhage, but Piersol [Footnote: Piersol: Pennsylvania Med. Jour., May, 1914, p. 625] finds that with perforation the peritoneal irritation may cause a rise of blood pressure, and he thinks that this sign may precede for several hours more positive signs of the accident.

As in other infections, the blood pressure will fall in scarlet fever; but if it suddenly rises, a kidney complication is to be looked for. The blood pressure always falls in diphtheria, and always falls in acute rheumatism; consequently, strenuous sweating measures in the treatment of rheumatism should not be used as soon as the blood pressure has become low.

Failing circulation in pneumonia, if accompanied by low blood pressure, requires different treatment from the failure of circulation in these cases when the blood pressure is high. Hence the relationship of the systolic to the diastolic pressure in pneumonia is of very great importance in deciding on the proper treatment. In one instance the blood pressure must be lowered; in the other, the heart must be stimulated.

While tobacco, in ordinary conditions, raises the blood pressure, after the heart has been seriously injured by the nicotin, the blood pressure is likely to be found lower, and such patients are quickly benefited by the withdrawal of the tobacco and the administration of digitalis.

Anemia almost invariably causes low blood pressure. Also in a patient who has hypotension without any distinct evidence of disease, especially if there has been any possible exposure to tuberculosis, that disease should be suspected and every test made to eliminate such a cause.

Serious cachexia, such as that caused by carcinoma or other growths, gives low blood pressure. Diabetes causes low blood pressure, provided there are no nephritis and no marked suprarenal stimulation.

Excessive use of alcohol, while tending to promote hypertension by the disturbances that it causes, may give, by causing a weak heart muscle, a permanent low blood pressure. A single large dose of alcohol always lowers the blood pressure.

Arteriosclerosis frequently reaches a stage when the blood pressure is low, and with atheroma of the arteries of the arms a true blood pressure is difficult to obtain. Addison's disease, or any other organic lesion of the suprarenals, will lower the pressure, while stimulation of the suprarenals increases the pressure. Any great drain on the system, whether from diabetes without nephritis, or from profuse diarrhea of any type, will cause hypotension. Occasionally a girl with chlorosis who is not menstruating may have an increased blood pressure. Many of the hemorrhagic or purpuric conditions will show a hypotension.

Meningitis in various forms may show a hypertension from cerebral and nervous irritation. Neurasthenic patients quite generally have hypotension, although occasionally with suprarenal disturbance they may have an increased tension.

In the hypotension of surgical shock and in shock during anesthesia, Henderson's findings [Footnote: Henderson: Am. Jour. Physiol., 1910, xxvii, 158.] that hyperoxygenation and insufficient carbon dioxid may be partially responsible for the condition should be remembered, and it has long been known that carbon dioxid congestion, as caused by laughing gas anesthesia, for instance, increases the blood pressure.

A systolic pressure of 110 mm. or lower in an adult should be considered hypotension, anything below 105 mm. calls for treatment, and a systolic pressure of 100 or lower in an adult calls for rest from all active duties.

These patients are weary, they have mental and physical tire, may get short breathed, may have palpitation of the heart, and often have headaches and dizziness from imperfect circulation in the head. There may be edemas of the legs and ankles toward night. If such patients have the systolic blood pressure raised even a small amount, or if the diastolic pressure, which is very low, is raised even a small amount, they immediately feel better.

If the kidneys are normal, they should have meat as part of their diet. If they are not nervous and irritable, coffee and tea should be allowed, except at the evening meal. While sleep may tend to lower pressure somewhat, these patients' hearts require a long bed rest; in other words, they should go to bed at an early hour. They should rise early, however, in the morning, and, as recommended by Goodman, [Footnote: Goodman: Am. Jour. Med. Sc., April, 1914, p. 503.] they should perform mild calisthenic exercises before dressing.

The increased muscle tone thus caused raises the blood pressure somewhat, and the great depression before breakfast is not experienced. These patients rely oil their morning coffee for bracing. If they have much indigestion at night which keeps them awake so that they do not get good comfortable rest, their largest meals should be the morning and noon meals, and the evening meal should be very light.

Pendent abdomens or ptosed abdominal organs should be held up by proper abdominal bandages or corsets.

If the bowels are constipated, only the vegetable laxatives should be used, if it drug is needed at all. Salines should not be allowed, or other cathartics which cause profuse watery discharges. If a brisk purge is required, castor oil is the best.

Plenty of fresh air, and mild exercises in the open air all tend to increase the pressure. Graded walking, climbing, or other more interesting exercises are advisable, as all tending to raise the pressure, provided that at no time are they carried to the point of exhaustion.

Forced feeding may be useful. Cool sponging in the morning, if there is proper reaction, is often of benefit. Iron may be indicated; bitter tonics may be indicated. Digitalis and strychnin are often of advantage. Caffein may be used as a drug as well as given in coffee and tea. Atropin may be of value in some forms of hypotension.

At times with a low systolic pressure, but a relatively high diastolic pressure, nitroglycerin is valuable.

More or less actite hypotension may occur in hot weather or with overheating, often termed heat exhaustion. Such patients should, if possible, go to a cooler region, whether to the seashore or to the mountains is unimportant. The treatment of dangerous sudden low blood pressure, as shock, will be discussed elsewhere.

PERICARDITIS

ACUTE PERICARDITIS

As this inflammation is generally secondary to some other condition, its treatment cannot be positively outlined. Furthermore, it is often a terminal condition, and in such instances the results of treatment are of necessity nil. The most frequent terminal cause is nephritis; other terminal causes are pulmonary tuberculosis, adjacent abscesses, cancer or other growth.

The most frequent infectious cause is rheumatism; other infectious causes are cerebrospinal fever, typhoid fever, acute miliary tuberculosis, pneumonia and Sepsis. Accidental causes are traumatism and an adjacent inflammation of the pleura.

The result of an inflammation of the pericardium may be a fibrous exudate, or an exudate which is both serous and fibrous, or one in which pus is present in considerable amount.

The onset of pericarditis may be more or less acute, or it may commence insidiously. For this reason, during severe illness, and especially in those diseases which are known to have pericarditis often as a sequence, frequent examination of the heart should be made as a routine procedure.

SYMPTOMS AND SIGNS

If there is pain or much aching in the cardiac region, it tends to disappear with the exudate, if such is to occur, in the same way as does the pain of pleurisy. If there is much exudate, the pressure on the heart of course increases, the cardiac dulness enlarges, dyspnea occurs and even perhaps later cyanosis. As the exudate accumulates, the patient must lie higher and higher in order that the fluid may gravitate to the lowest part of the sac and give the heart the greatest ability to work. Reflex pain may occur from disturbances of the pneumogastric nerve, or from the weight and pressure of the enlarged and heavy pericardium. Reflex vomiting may be a troublesome and distressing symptom.

Acute pericarditis occurring in rheumatism, in acute infections, and from simple injuries tends to recovery. In dry pericarditis with serious adhesions, or if adhesions occur as a sequence of acute pericarditis, the future prognosis is bad, as myocarditis may develop and sudden death or acute dilatation may occur. As stated above, if pericarditis develops during the progress of chronic disease, such as interstitial nephritis, or during sepsis, or from abscesses or growths in the region of the pericardium, the prognosis is bad.

TREATMENT OF ACUTE PERICARDITIS

In acute pericarditis, absolute mental as well as physical rest is essential. Even if the patient does not appear to be seriously ill and has not much fever, he should not be allowed to have visitors, to discuss business matters, or to carry on any conversation, however little exciting. Anything which increases the heart beat increases the irritation of the inflamed surfaces of the pericardium. He should not be allowed to sit up, either to eat or to attend to the calls of Nature. These rules are imperative, and when they are followed the pain is less, the heart beats less rapidly, is less hampered by pressure from whatever exudate may be present, and the adhesions which are liable to form will be less in amount and less serious for the future work of the heart.

The treatment, of course, depends largely on the cause of the pericarditis, as, if the cause is one of those just enumerated in which the prognosis is dire, any treatment directed toward the pericardial inflammation is almost useless. The periearditis under these conditions will be more or less benefited, if at all affected, by the treatment directed toward the cause.

The indications for treatment in all other instances are:

1. To attempt to abort the inflammation.

2. To stop the pain.

3. To limit, if possible, the amount of exudate, and to diminish the exudate already present.

4. To diminish the rapidity of the heart and to strengthen it.

1. Abortive Treatment.—For many years bloodletting was considered of the greatest importance in the early treatment of this disease; but owing to the fact that, except from traumatism, pericarditis rarely occurs except as a sequela of acute disease after the patient has been sick along time, or as a terminal condition in a patient who has long been chronically diseased and therefore has already lost more or less strength, venesection has been nearly abandoned. Leeches may be used over the region of the pericardium, and cups are sometimes used. Dry cupping is more frequently used. These measures sometimes seem to reduce the inflammation, and certainly often relieve pain, but the most valuable local treatment is cold, which may be applied either in the form of an ice bag or by a small coil through which ice water is caused to flow by siphonage. Cold may be applied more or less continuously, depending on the sensations of the patient. The bag or ice cap must not be overfilled and must not be heavy, as the patient often cannot stand pressure over the pericardium. Sometimes the relief from pain and the diminution of the number of the heart beats is marked, and for this reason alone the cardiac inflammation may be inhibited. If cold applications are not tolerated by the patient (and they often are not in children) warm applications may be used, such as an electric pad or cloths wrung out of hot water and covered with oiled silk, and the pain will often be relieved thus. While hot applications would not tend to abort the inflammation, they probably do not tend to promote it.

A diminished diet, of small amount at a time, and such purging as the patient's strength will allow are essential in attempting to hasten recovery.

Just what can be done locally or generally to combat the inflammation actively must depend on the cause. When the inflammation occurs as a complication of acute rheumatism, it has been suggested that salicylates, which arc not inhibiting rheumatism and may be depressant to the heart, should be stopped if they are being administered; but if the salicylates are apparently improving the inflammation in the joints, pericarditis would not contraindicate their continued use. Except in large doses, salicylates probably do not depress the heart. In pericarditis it is perhaps well always to administer an alkali in some form unless otherwise contraindicated, whether or not the cause is rheumatism. A diminished alkalinity of the blood would always increase the likelihood of an augmented amount of pericardial or endocardial inflammation. The blood must be kept strongly alkaline. It is possible that one of the reasons why pericarditis or endocarditis occurs so frequently in serious prolonged fevers is that the patient has not eaten enough cereals or other carbohydrates, and the system has become more or less endangered by acidosis. Carbohydrate starvation is inexcusable with our present understanding of the danger from acideinia, and even from a diminished amount of alkalies in the blood.

The cause of pericarditis being so varied, any anti-toxin treatment or any vaccine treatment could be indicated only if the cause of the inflammation rendered the serum or vaccine advisable.

2. Stopping the Pain.—Nowhere else in the body should pain be so speedily combated as when it occurs in the region of the heart. Morphin, with or without atropin, as deemed best, should be administered hypodermically in the amount and with the frequency necessary to stop the pain and quiet the restlessness. As stated above, the frequent need for morphin may be prevented by use of the ice bag. Morphin might even be considered an abortive treatment, as nothing tends so much to inhibit this inflammation as the quietude of the heart caused by the absence of pain, the production of sleep and the prevention of restlessness, muscle twitching and muscle movements. The more quiet the patient is, the more quiet is the heart.

If for any reason morphin is contraindicated, and if pain is not a symptom, the patient's nerves may be quieted and rest may be given by sodium bromid, or by veronal-sodium, the dose of the former being 2 gm. (30 grains) two or three times in twenty-four hours, according to its action and the necessity for it, and the dose of the latter 0.2 gm. (3 grains) once in six hours, if deemed necessary.

Especially if there are cerebral symptoms, as typically presented in cerebrospinal meningitis, and especially if the arterial tension is low, the subcutaneous administration of an aseptic ergot will quiet the central nervous system, increase the blood pressure, quiet the heart, and prolong the action of a single dose of morphin. It is the best plan to administer ergot deep into the muscles, with the deltoid as the place of choice. If the skin is properly cleansed, the syringe clean and the preparation of the drug aseptic, no inflammation or abscess will ever occur. If there is any painful swelling, a wet alcohol dressing to the part will soon relieve it. The frequence with which ergot should be so administered depends on the results and the indications. Once in twelve hours for several doses is generally the best method for its use.

3. The Exudate.—When a fluid exudate into the pericardium has occurred from inflammation that is, when it is not an exudate from disturbed kidneys or circulation—it will continue to increase to some extent in spite of any treatment. Just how much this exudate may be prevented by the use of small blisters over or around the heart, and just how much watery stools and diuresis may prevent the advance of the exudate is difficult to determine. Small blisters, properly applied, have many times seemed to be the determining factor in stopping the increase in the fluid, or to have been the starting cause of the resorption of the exudate.

The amount of purging that should be caused by saline cathartics such as sodium sulphate (Glauber salt), potassium and sodium tartrate (Rochelle salt), or the official compound jalap powder cannot be declared dogmatically. Saline purging should be governed by the character of the circulation. If the heart is strong, the pulse not weak, and the blood pressure good, nothing is more valuable in this condition. Portal depletion is of great advantage, especially if the amount of liquid ingested is kept as low as possible, so that the blood vessels may become thirsty and thus tend to absorb an exudate wherever they find it. Much harm has been done, however, and death has been caused by saline purgatives in endeavoring to relieve edemas from a failing heart or to prevent a uremia from kidney inflammation. The depression following such purging is often serious. If the circulation is weak, dependence should be placed on purgation by some of the simple vegetable cathartics or a small dose of calomel. While it is advisable to give a saline in concentrated solution, it should not be so strong as to cause vomiting. With our better understanding of magnesium absorption and the depressant effect of magnesium on the nervous system, magnesium salts should not be used in serious conditions.

Diuretics often do not act well when most needed. The simplest diuretic is potassium citrate, given in wintergreen or peppermint water, in doses of 2 gm. (30 grains), three or four tunes in twenty-four hours. One or more of the vegetable, nonirritant diuretics may be tried if preferred. If the sickness preceding the pericarditis was not a long fever, and the heart muscle is considered in good condition, digitalis in small doses may be the best possible diuretic. Incidentally it will slow the heart, if there is not much elevation of temperature, and will give some cardiac rest.

Although the patient's diet should be limited in bulk, and especially in amount of liquids, good nutrition should soon be given. Systemic weakness certainly tends to increase the exudate; systemic strength aids in absorption of the exudate.

Iron is early indicated, and nothing is better than 5 drops of the tincture of chlorid of iron in a little lemonade or orangeade, administered once in eight hours.

If the exudate tends to decrease, it perhaps may be hastened by the local application of tincture of iodin over the cardiac region. Also the administration of small doses of an iodid, as 0.3 gm. (5 grains) of sodium iodid, given in plenty of water three times a day, is useful. An iodid circulating in the blood seems to aid absorption. It has long been believed that iodin in the blood tends to promote absorption of thickened, left-over material from exudates, and to prevent the formation of strong fibrous adhesions. Until our knowledge is more exact in this matter, it is advisable to use iodid as suggested. If the above-named dose is not tolerated, less should be given.

If in spite of all the therapeutic measures suggested, the fluid increases and the pericardium becomes more distended and the heart's action more labored, paracentesis must be done. The point at which the aspirating needle should be inserted into the pericardium depends somewhat on the conditions in each individual case. It is often best to insert an exploratory needle first. This will determine the fluidity and character of the exudate. If pus is found, a more radical surgical procedure than simple paracentesis must be done immediately. The point of puncture for aspiration most frequently chosen is in the fourth or fifth intercostal space, about an inch to the left of the sternal margin. Paracentesis is also often done in the region of the normal apex beat. The position of the patient is determined by his dyspnea; he should lie in the position most comfortable for him. The fluid should be withdrawn slowly and the pulse carefully watched. The withdrawal of a small amount of fluid may later seem to be the starting cause of resorption of the rest of the fluid. On the other hand, it may often be not of more value than the simple removal of the immediate pressure, the fluid may again accumulate, and more radical surgery must be performed.

4. To Strengthen the Heart.—Most of the methods of meeting this indication have already been stated, namely, absolute rest; absolute quiet; the use of the bed pan; any movement that must be made should be deliberate; the nurse and other attendants must be quiet; necessary conversation must be brief, and every method must be used to quiet and prevent the heart's action from becoming rapid. The food taken should be small in amount and nonstimulating; that is, no tea or coffee should be given, and nothing too hot or too cold. Movements of the bowels should be caused with the least possible general disturbance. If the patient does not sleep, he must be made to sleep. The whole body and the nervous system must have periods of rest. If the heart is very weak, small closes of morphin may be used. If the heart is not weak, bromids or chloral may be given. If the blood pressure is high, such hypnotics will lower it, or if the heart is strong and the condition does not contraindicate it, aconite may be used in small doses, for a day or two, unless the fever is high and it seems advisable to use one of the coal-tar antipyretics, which reduce the blood tension and the heart activity.

As stated above, pain must not be allowed. Sometimes, when the heart has not been injured by prolonged fever, digitalis in small doses may slow the heart and act for good.

Convalescence.—The convalescence should be prolonged as in any other cardiac inflammation. The patient should be given more and more nourishing food, and the iron tonic may be changed to a capsule containing 0.05 gm. of quinin and 0.05 gm. of reduced iron, three times a day.

It is a question as to when patients convalescent from pericarditis should be permitted exercise. It has been thought that gentle movements and possibly exercise, sooner than theoretically justified, might cause the heart to beat a little more actively and possibly prevent the formation of tight adhesions between the two layers of the pericardium. Whether such activity of the heart will prevent adhesions is something that has not been determined.

The small doses of sodium iodid, perhaps 0.2 gm. (3 grains) two or three times a day, should be continued for some time. Iodid in this dosage does no harm and may do a great deal of good.

ADHERENT PERICARDITIS

Following dry pericarditis or pericarditis with an exudate, especially when the exudate is fibrinous in character, the fibrous substance which is not absorbed or resorbed may develop into connective tissue, and the two pericardial surfaces become permanently grown together, causing the so-called adherent pericarditis. These adhesions between the two surfaces of the pericardium may be general throughout the entire pericardial sac, or they may be limited to some one or more parts of the pericardium. Perhaps one of the most frequent points of adhesion is the anterior part of the pericardium, while the apex is the part most likely to be free, even when other parts of the pericardium have grown together. This freedom of the apex is probably due to the constant and more extensive motion of the apical portion of the heart, and is the reason that it has been suggested, as referred to under acute pericarditis, that, other conditions not contraindicating, the patient may be allowed to move about a little during convalescence to cause the heart to beat more actively. Sometimes the surfaces of the pericardium are not closely adherent to each other, but bands of adhesion stretch from one surface to the other.

After adhesions have taken place between the two layers of the pericardium, the action of the heart is impaired, serious interference with the cardiac action may develop, and sudden death may occur. If the heart is given all the rest possible during the acute phase of the disease, there will be less likelihood of the surfaces becoming so irritated that adhesions readily form. Anything which permits complete absorption and resorption of tile exudate will tend to prevent these hampering adhesions. If the adhesions are such as to cause irregular heart, recurrent pain and the danger of sudden death, surgical help has been suggested. This surgical procedure is to remove a portion of the ribs, perhaps of the third, fourth and fifth, to allow the heart more freedom of action to compensate for the impairment of its activity from the adhesions. Such an operation was first suggested by Brauer of Heidelberg in 1902.

The question of the best method of producing anesthesia in this condition of the heart is a serious one. A patient might die during the anesthesia; but he might also die at any time from cardiac spasm. In certain instances, in adults, local anesthesia might be sufficient. Pain reflexes, however, would be serious. Such an operation would be indicated when the apex is fixed so that there is a constant sensation of hugging of the heart at the fourth and fifth ribs, with paroxysms of pain and cardiac weakness.

MYOCARDIAL DISTURBANCES

While the myocardium is the most important muscle structure of the body, it has but recently been studied carefully or well understood clinically or pathologically. A heart was "hypertrophied" or "dilated" or perhaps "fatty." It suffered from "pain," "angina pectoris," from some "serious weakness" or from "coronary disease," and that ended the pathology and the clinical diagnosis. This is the age of heart defects; no one can understand a patient's condition now, whatever ails him, without studying his heart. No one can treat a patient properly now without considering the management of the circulation. No one should administer a drug now without considering what it will do to the patient's heart.

Although we are scientifically interested in the administration of specific treatments, antitoxins and vaccines; although we have a better understanding of food values, and order diets with more careful consideration of the exact needs of the individual, and although we are using various physical methods to promote elimination of toxins, poisons and products of metabolism, we have until lately forgotten the physical fact that one thirteenth of the weight of a normal adult is blood. A man who weighs 170 pounds has 13 pounds of blood. This proportion is not true in the obese, and is not true in children. Whether the person is sick in bed, miserable though up and about, or beginning to feel the first sensations of slight incapacity for his life work, his ability properly to circulate this one thirteenth of his weight through the various arterial and venous channels and capillary tracts must, with the increasing tension and speed of our lives, be taken into consideration.

The more and more frequently repeated statements that the operation was successfully performed but that the patient died of shock, and that the typhoid fever and the pneumonia were being successfully combated, but that the patient died of heart failure, together with the increase in arteriosclerosis, cardiac disturbances and renal disease, emphatically present the necessity of more carefully studying the circulation. A better understanding and the constant study of the blood pressure shows nothing but the necessity of the age. The unwillingness of the patient to suffer pain, even for a few minutes, without some narcotic, generally a cardiac debilitating drug, means that, if he is a sufferer from chronic or recurrent pain, he has taken a great deal of medicine which has done his heart no good. Repeated high tension of life raises the blood pressure and puts more work on the heart. Therefore the heart is found weary, if not actually degenerated, when any serious accident, medical or surgical, happens to the patient.

The requirements of the age have, then, necessitated that the heart be more carefully studied, and therefore the heart strength and its disturbances are better understood. The mere determination as to where the apex beat is located, and as to what murmurs may be present is not sufficient; we must attempt to determine the probable condition of the myocardium. The following conditions are recognized: (1) acute myocarditis, (2) chronic myocarditis (fibrosis, cardiosclerosis), (3) fatty degeneration, and (4) fatty heart.

ACUTE MYOCARDITIS

Probably most acute infections cause more or less myocarditis, depending on their intensity and their prolongation. This disturbance of the heart is often unrecognized, and has been simply referred to as "the heart growing weaker from the fever process." The acute infections most likely to cause a myocarditis are rheumatism, influenza, sepsis, cerebrospinal meningitis, diphtheria, typhoid fever, scarlet fever, and mouth and throat infections. It is probably rare when acute endocarditis occurs that more or less myocarditis is not present. The acute myocarditis may develop some fatty degeneration, and with this softening and weakening of the heart muscle acute dilatation readily occurs, which may be a cause of sudden death, or, if less serious, may be the cause of prolonged disability, if the heart ever recovers its original size and strength.

The symptoms are often indefinite, and the diagnosis of the condition hardly possible. It may be taken for granted, however, that hardly any serious illness can long continue without cardiac muscle disturbance. If endocarditis is present, soft systolic murmurs soon appear. With the acute myocarditis developing, the apex beat is less positive, less accentuated, and later it becomes diffuse and even feeble. The closure of the aortic valve is less typically sharp, showing that the blood vessels are not so thoroughly filled. The peripheral circulation is not so active, the blood pressure falls, and the heart becomes more rapid, especially on the least exertion. All of these signs indicate myocardial weakness.

The treatment of this condition is largely preventive. It should be well recognized that prolonged high fever, prolonged insufficient or improper nutrition, prolonged acute pain, and especially prolonged septic processes will always cause myocardial degeneration. It should be recognized that after ether and chloroform anesthesia, especially after chloroform, the heart muscle may be disturbed and the tonicity be lost. Therefore after anesthesia, after operations, and after all illnesses which have lasted more than a few days, the convalescence of the patient must be more or less deliberate. Sudden rising, sudden erect posture, the exertion of walking too early, going up stairs too early or taking moderate, and later severe exercise too early, may cause dilatation of the heart muscle that has become weakened by acute myocarditis. If acute myocarditis is believed or known to be present, cardiac tonics such as digitalis should not be given; large doses of strychnin should not be given; vasocontractors such as ergot should not be given; large amounts of food or large bulks of liquid should not be taken into the stomach at one time; in fact, unless there is some special indication, the twenty-four hour amount of fluid should be diminished. The surface circulation and the muscle circulation should be improved by such cold or warm water applications as the disease or condition calls for. Massage should be early inaugurated to promote the return circulation. The heart should be treated as though it were the frailest of Venetian glass and would crack with the least rough handling, or even with a rapid change of temperature, great cold or too much heat. A prolonged, tedious convalescence, with the return to activity so graded as to give the heart no strain, and to keep its work always just below what it is able to do, will often mean return to perfect strength and health.

No cardiac debilitating drug should be administered when myocarditis has been surmised or diagnosed. The safest hypnotic, if one is needed, is morphin in small doses. If there are weakening perspirations, atropin should be given, especially as it is also a circulatory stimulant. Calcium in almost any form seems to be of value in the majority of heart conditions. It is a sedative to the nervous system, and is certainly indicated in acute myocarditis. Calcium lactate is perhaps the best salt to administer, in doses of 0.25 gm. (4 grains), three or four times in twenty-four hours. Calcium glycerophosphate may be used, in powder form or in capsule, in doses of 0.30 gm. (5 grains) three or four times in twenty-four hours; or lime-water may be given.

An exact prognosis of this inflammation is impossible. We do not know how far an acute myocarditis may progress and entire recovery take place; we do not know how slight a myocarditis may cause serious symptoms. Clinically we know that many patients after serious illness never again have perfect circulatory strength. Other patients almost die of heart failure and yet apparently absolutely recover their ability to do hard physical work.

CHRONIC MYOCARDITIS: FIBROUS

Chronic myocarditis may develop on an acute myocarditis, but is generally a slowly progressive chronic process from the beginning; it occurs mostly in persons past middle life, and as a rule is not primarily associated with rheumatism or valvular disease of the heart. Perhaps generally the term "chronic myocarditis" is incorrect, as a real inflammatory condition is not present and has not been present; it is really a degenerative process with the development of connective tissue, a fibrosis and more or less hardening of the arterioles, a cardiosclerosis. In many instances this fibrosis is associated with fat deposits or fatty degeneration. The disease is often caused by a narrowing or obstruction or calcareous degeneration of the coronary arteries, thus diminishing the blood supply to the heart muscle. This chronic myocardial degeneration is often a part of the general arteriosclerosis, and is an important factor in what is termed cardiovascular-renal disease. In simple chronic renal diseases the heart first normally hypertrophies to overcome the increased blood tension and increased resistance.

The principal causes of this degeneration are normal old age, or premature age caused by various conditions. In other words, anything which hastens arteriosclerosis will cause myocardial degeneration. The causes recognized as most frequently producing this condition are syphilis; gout; repeated attacks of rheumatism; excess in the use of alcohol (meaning repeated daily too large amounts, as well as actual dipsomania); the overuse of tobacco; excess in drinking tea or coffee; general overeating, and excessive eating of meat in particular, if the organs of elimination do not work perfectly and if such eating causes or allows putrefactive changes in the intestines; and progressive, prolonged wasting diseases, such as tuberculosis and cancer. It has also seemed in some cases that the only cause was excessive, hard physical labor, including excessive athletic work, and in other cases that prolonged anxiety and worry have been causes of cardiac degeneration and actual cardiac failure. Prolonged absorption of toxins from mouth and tonsil infections may be a not infrequent cause.

These myocardial changes are sometimes associated with chronic pericarditis and chronic endocarditis, and may accompany or follow valvular disease of the heart. Failure of compensation in valvular disease and dilatation of the heart are sequences which occur sooner or later.

SYMPTOMS AND SIGNS

The symptoms of chronic myocardial degeneration are progressive weakness, slight at first, noticeable on exertion (and what was not considered exertion becomes such), as evidenced by slight palpitation, slight shortness of breath, leg weariness and mental tire. The heart frequently becomes more rapid, not only with exertion and change of position to the erect, but even after eating. Slight cardiac stimulants, as coffee, affect the heart more than previously; there is some sleeplessness, more or less troublesome, and more or less indigestion. There may be mental irritability and some mental deterioration, as shown in various ways. There are likely to be slight edemas of the lower extremities toward night. The amount of urine may diminish. A previously high blood pressure becomes lower. The pulse may be occasionally intermittent, and later actually irregular.

The physical signs often show an enlargement of the heart, with increased activity at first, from irritability of the heart and a lack of perfect coordination; later the heart may show typical signs of weakness. Not infrequently a heart suffering from fibrosis acts perfectly until some sudden exertion, as lifting, running or serious illness causes it suddenly to become weak. Such a heart rarely regains its former strength. This occurs frequently to those who have supposed themselves to be in perfect physical health. Some sudden strain which they have previously been able to endure without injury, such as carrying a weight upstairs, cranking a refractory engine, pumping up a series of tires, or walking rapidly with a younger or more active companion, will suddenly give cardiac distress signals, serious exhaustion and more or less lengthy prostration, perhaps for an hour or so, or perhaps for several days. Permanent cardiac weakness may follow, or compensation may again occur, to be more easily broken later. Slight cardiac pains and sensations referred to the cardiac region become frequent. Disliking to lie on the left side, when previously the patient has been able to sleep on this side without discomfort, is an evidence of cardiac disturbance. There may be no real pains, but the patient becomes conscious of his heart, perhaps for the first time in his life. This alone is an indication of coming trouble.

If these signs and symptoms develop late in life, or at any age with other symptoms of sclerosis or senility, little can be done therapeutically except to afford temporary relief and to prevent the occurrence of acute attacks of cardiac distress or dyspnea. If the disturbance is really due to chronic cardiac degeneration, the sooner the patient learns that his ability is restricted, that his life is narrowed, the better for his future.

MANAGEMENT

The advice he should receive is well understood: to avoid physical efforts; to avoid mental tire; to avoid overeating or overdrinking of any foods or liquids; to reduce or abstain from alcohol, coffee, tea and tobacco, depending on what seems advisable in the individual case; to reduce the amount of meat eaten, especially if there is intestinal indigestion; to relieve intestinal indigestion; to cause free daily movements of the bowels; to abstain from any food which tends to cause gastric or intestinal flatulence; to abstain from such foods as contain nucleins, if the patient is gouty; to take frequent warm baths (not too hot) to promote the secretions and the circulation in the skin, and to take such daily exercise as seems advisable. If the patient cannot take exercise, simple calisthenics or massage should be instituted.

Whether nitroglycerin or other nitrite is advisable depends on the peripheral blood pressure. If the blood pressure is low, or not higher than is best for the patient, such treatment would be inadvisable. If, from the supposed cause, iodid seems to be indicated, it should be given in small doses and continued for some time. It is often wise, however, to give small doses, as 0.10 or 0.20 gm. (2 or 3 grains) once or twice in twenty-four hours, for a long period, to any patient who leas fibrosis or selerosis in any form. Iodid tends to prevent the progress of connective tissue formation. It is quite possible that some of its value is in activating a sluggish or imperfectly acting thyroid gland. If the patient is old, his thyroid is subinvoluting, and a little more of its activity will be of advantage. Many diseases which cause chronic myocarditis also cause, later, subactivity of the thyroid. Thyroid extract may be indicated if the patient is obese.

If, in spite of this management and treatment, the patient has cardiac asthma attacks, with or without pain, especially if there are pendent edemas, the question arises as to whether or not digitalis should be given. In such cases one cannot tell without trying whether digitalis will be of benefit or will cause more discomfort. 11 small dose of an active preparation should be given at first twice in twenty-four hours, and after a week once in twenty-four hours, its action being carefully watched and the decision as to whether the dose is too large or too small arrived at. It may do a great amount of good; it can cause increased cardiac pains. If used carefully and stopped when it appears not to be acting well, it will do no harm.

Chilling of the surface of the body should be avoided; sudden cold or sustained severe cold, which increases the contraction of the peripheral blood vessels and puts more strain on the heart muscle, is to be avoided if possible. More hours in bed at night and lying down after the heavier meals of the day will tend to give the heart the kind of rest it needs. Also complete rest for one day a week, or a rest of several days at a time, and a rest, both mental and physical, with such walking, golfing or riding as seems advisable, for at least one month every year, will prolong the lives of these patients, and may make an imperfect heart act well for months and years. If the patient is anemic he should, of course, receive some nonastringent iron; a. tablet of saccharated ferric oxid (Eisenzucker), in small doses, 0.20 gm. (3 grains), once or twice in twenty-four hours, is sufficient.

The prognosis of a case diagnosed as chronic myocarditis or chronic degeneration of the heart is doubtful, as one cannot tell until several weeks or months of observation whether this particular heart also has fatty degeneration or not. If there is fatty degeneration, the prognosis is bad. If there is no serious fatty degeneration, the patient, with the modified life outlined, may live for a long time. Acute dilatation from any serious strain on the heart may occur, and if there is fatty degeneration it is liable to occur at any time. Attacks of cardiac asthma are always serious, and always damage the heart a little more.

FATTY DEGENERATION

Fatty degeneration of the heart muscle may be caused by acute poisoning (as phosphorus, arsenic, etc.), by serious infections, or it may follow fibrosis of the heart or coronary artery disease. The symptoms are those of serious circulatory weaicnens, which does not seem to improve under any ordinary management. It is difficult, if the heart is enlarged, to determine whether there is more or less serious acute dilatation or whether the heart muscle has suffered fatty degenration.

The treatment of such a patient requires the best of judgment as to the amount of food and liquid that should be given, the regulation of the administration of laxatives, the sponging of the body, the means of producing sleep if there is insomnia, how much reading, conversation or amusements should be allowed, how much stimulation by stryclmin or other stimulating drug should be given, and whether or not very small doses of digitalis should he tried. These are all matters for individualizing, and for the best medical judgment which we are called on to give. How much repair can take place in a heart muscle when fatty degeneration has started we do not know. Such treatment will give the heart the only chance it has to recuperate, but the prognosis is bad.

FATTY HEART

The cause of deposits of fat around the heart or in between its chambers is the same as the cause of general obesity. These patients are likely to be obese, or at least to have large abdomens with large deposits of fat around the abdomen. This fat in itself will interfere somewhat with abdominal respiration. This tends to cause dyspnea, and the heart tends to be disturbed from these causes, if much fat is not really in the pericardium. The symptoms are those of imperfect heart action; the patient is dyspneic on exertion or in leaning over, the heart acts rapidly on such exertion, the patient puffs, perspires easily, and becomes leg weary, sedentary in his habits, and more or less incapacitated for work. He may not be a large eater; if he is, and his eating habit is corrected, the prognosis is better than if he is putting on weight in spite of eating sparingly.

The general treatment is that for obesity, and if the heart muscle is intact, various depletion methods may be inaugurated. More and more exercise, sweatings from Turkish baths, electric-light baths, body baking, vigorous massage and more or less purging are all valuable. Anything which reduces the general weight will help the heart. The prognosis is often good.

ENDOCARDITIS

It should be understood that especially in acute conditions a positive separation of endocarditis from myocarditis is incorrect. Acute endocarditis can probably not occur without some inyocarditis, and myocarditis probably does not occur without some endocardial disturbance and perhaps some pericardial irritation. This is especially true in endocarditis which occurs during any acute infection, even in rheumatism. The greater the amount of pericarditis, the more serious is the acute condition. The greater the amount of myocarditis, the more doubtful is the heart strength in the near future. The greater the amount of endocarditis, the greater the doubt of freedom from future permanent valvular lesions.

Endocarditis may be divided into: acute mild (simple) endocarditis, acute malignant (ulcerative, infective) endocarditis, chronic endocarditis and valvular disease.

ACUTE MILD ENDOCARDITIS

This inflammation of the endocardium is generally confined to the region of the valves, and the valves most frequently so inflamed are the mitral and aortic. There may be a slight inflammation or actual ulceration and loss of tissue. Vegetations more or less constantly occur on the inflamed surfaces, with more or less danger of particles becoming loosened and moving free in the blood stream, causing embolic obstruction in different parts of the body. There is also more or less probability of serious adhesions or contractions occurring from the healing of the ulcerated surfaces. The future health and welfare of the valves depend on the fact that the inflammation has healed without contractions or adhesions.

It is often difficult to decide when acute endocarditis has developed; but with the knowledge that the endocardium often becomes inflamed during almost any of the acute infections, the physician should repeatedly examine the heart for murmurs, for muffled closure of the valves, or for other evidences of endocarditis or myocarditis during the acute infective process.

It has been shown positively that acute endocarditis is due to micro-organisms, generally streptococci, staphylococci or pneumococci, and, more frequently than once believed, gonococci. The most frequent causes are acute rheumatic fever, diphtheria, pneumonia, cerebrospinal meningitis, scarlet fever, erysipelas, influenza, chorea, gonorrhea, sepsis and typhoid fever. It may also follow a follicular tonsillitis or some infection of the mouth or throat with or without arthritis. Tuberculosis may also occasionally cause an endocarditis. Organisms may be found in a terminal simple endocarditis due to a chronic disease, as tuberculosis or cancer; such inflammations may have been caused by circulating toxins.

It will be noticed by the foregoing classification that the terms "mild" and "malignant" endocarditis are used. The purpose is to convey the fact that there may be no etiologic distinction between the two forms, and it is impossible to decide clinically in the beginning of an endocardial inflammation which form is present. In the malignant form the infection is probably more serious or the infective germs are more active, the ulcerations deeper, and the likelihood of emboli and the seriousness of such embolic infarcts more serious and more dangerous. The differences in inflammation in the two cases is really one of degree, and the classification is made to coincide with this probable fact. it is, of course, clinically recognized that endocarditis following certain diseases, especially rheumatism, is of the simple or mild type, while that termed ulcerative endocarditis may occur apparently as a primary or general infection, and the causative bacteria, as a rule, are readily discovered in the blood. The Streptococcus viridans is one of the most dangerous of these bacteria.

A SECONDARY AFFECTION

Mild endocarditis is rarely a primary affection, and is almost invariably secondary to one of the diseases named above. Nearly 75 percent of secondary endocarditis occurs as a complication of acute articular rheumatism and chorea, or subsequently. On the other hand, about 40 percent of all patients with acute articular rheumatism develop endocarditis, sometimes perhaps so mild as to be hardly discoverable. This complication is most likely to occur during the second or third week of rheumatic fever. It is not sufficiently recognized that a subacute arthritis, recurring tonsillitis, open and concealed infections in the mouth, and even a condition of the system with acute, changeable and varying joint and muscle pains may all develop a mild endocarditis, even with subsequent valvular lesions. Therefore in all of these conditions the decision can be made only as to how much rest the patient must have or how serious the condition is to be considered by careful examination of the heart in every instance.

Children are more liable than adults to this complication, especially with rheumatism. Therefore, acute mild endocarditis with future valvular lesions occurs most frequently during childhood and adolescence, and if one attack has occurred, a subsequent infection, especially of rheumatism, is liable to cause another acute endocarditis.

PATHOLOGY

The part of the heart most affected is the part which has the most work to do—the left side of the heart—and of this side the left ventricle and therefore the mitral and aortic valves; the most frequent valve to be inflamed and to stiffer permanent disability is the a mitral valve, the valve which in its inflamed condition is subjected to the greatest amount of pressure and therefore irritation. Not infrequently soft systolic murmurs are heard at the pulmonary and tricuspid valves during acute endocarditis. It is rare, however, that these valves are so affected during childhood or adult life as to be permanently disabled.

Whether a diminished alkalinity of the blood in rheumatism has anything to do with the cause of the frequent complication of endocarditis has not been determined. Whether the administration of alkalies to the point of increasing the alkalinity of the blood is any protection against the complication of endocarditis has also not been positively demonstrated, although clinically such treatment is believed by a large number of practitioners to be wise.

A chronic endocarditis with permanent lesions of the valves may become an acute inflammation with an infectious provocation.

It has been shown that even in a few hours after endocarditis has started, little vegetations composed of fibrin, with white blood cells, red blood pigment and platelets, may develop. Practically in all instances such vegetations develop, and later become more or less organized into connective tissue. These little vegetations, generally minute, perhaps not exceeding 4 mm. in height, are irregular in contour like a wart. Some of these may have small pedicles, and as such, of course, are more likely to become loosened and fly off into the blood stream. It is of interest to note that these little vegetations are more likely to be on the left side of the heart than the right; on the valves than any other part, and on the mitral valve than on the aortic. The consequence is a more frequent permanent disability of the valves of the left side of the heart, and of these more frequently the mitral. Although these little vegetations and excrescences sooner or later become mostly connective tissue, still fibrin and white blood cells may form thin layers over them, more or less permanent. In this fibrin are frequently found bacteria, even when there has been no recent acute inflammation. The deeper layers of the endocardium during acute inflammation may become infiltrated with young cells, with resultant softening and destruction of the intercellular substance. This softening and some swelling of the lower layers of the endocardium allow the pushing up of these extravasated blood cells which, being covered with fibrin, makes the little vegetations above described; and as just stated, the fibrin may form a more or less permanent cap. If this cap is disintegrated or lost and the cells under it washed away in the blood stream, ulceration takes place, which may be more or less serious, even to the perforation of a valve or actual erosion of one of its cusps, and the parts of the valves most seriously affected are the parts which strike against each other on closure; as previously stated, the parts subjected to the greatest strain and the greatest amount of friction during the inflammation are the parts most seriously affected afterward.

If a perforation has occurred, it may make a permanent leak. If an erosion of the edge of the valve has occurred, it may make permanent insufficient closure. If the valve has become thickened and stiffened during the cicatricial healing, it may not only be incompetent, but may not open perfectly, and a narrowed orifice may be the consequence. During the healing of these granulating ulcers there may be thickening of the part or shrinking of the tissue, and the valve may become shortened by adhesion to the wall, or the cusps of the valve may adhere together so that the valve becomes permanently unable to open properly or to close properly, or to do either.

Not infrequently and probably more frequently than we recognize, recovery without any of the pathologic lesions just described follows mild endocarditis. The occurrence of simple endocarditis is undoubtedly frequent during acute disease, and is unrecognized because there are no lesions of the heart at the time or subsequently; but valvular lesions only too frequently follow the endocarditis which occurs with rheumatism. Occasionally the ulcerations become serious, and ulcerative endocarditis or malignant endocarditis develops on the mild inflammation. In this form the little vegetations are liable to become loosened, fly off into the blood stream, and cause emboli in different parts of the body.

Recently Fraenkel [Footnote: Fraenkel: Beitr. z. path. Anat. u. z. allg. Path., 1912, iii, 597.] concluded that the microscopic nodules which occur in endocarditis in the myocardium, and which consist of the several varieties of white blood corpuscles first referred to by Aschoff in 1904, are characteristic only of acute rheumatism. Fraenkel found these nodules in the myocardium in a case of chorea, showing the close relationship between it and rheumatism.

While repeated careful examination of the heart during acute infections will generally show signs of endocarditis if it is present, even if there are no subjective symptoms, the disease may be so insidious as not to be noted until a valvular lesion occurs. Often, however, during the course of the disease, especially in rheumatism, there is a slight increase in fever and there is a discomfort complained of in the region of the heart, frequently accompanied by slight dyspnea. Real pain is seldom present unless the pericardium is affected. If the myocardium is much inflamed at the same time, the heart becomes more rapid and the blood tension lowered, and the apex beat diminished in intensity and perhaps not palpable. If there is pain, with or without pericarditis, it is often referred to the epigastrium, especially in children. The patient is often nervous, restless and sleepless. In simple endocarditis emboli rarely occur. If they do, of course the signs will be in the part in which the infarct occurs. Besides the diminished intensity of the apex beat and its greater diffusion, the valve sounds may be muffled, and sooner or later there may be systolic murmurs over the different orifices. Of course systolic murmurs may be due to a disturbed condition of the blood, but if they occur with the above-mentioned symptoms and signs, endocarditis should be diagnosed. If the heart becomes seriously weak and the patient suffers much dyspnea, myocarditis should be known to be present with the endocarditis. If there is a diastolic murmur, there can be no question of serious endocarditis having occurred. Unexplainable palpation during acute illness liar been thought to be a distinct symptom of endocarditis.

TREATMENT OF ENDOCARDITIS

As mild endocarditis rarely occurs primarily but is almost always secondary to some acute disease, its immediate treatment is only a slight modification of that of the disease which is causing it. A complication which is so frequent should always be expected, and consequently warded off or prevented, if possible. Knowledge of the diseases which are most liable to cause endocarditis makes frequent heart examinations a necessity, to note when it arrives. While an extra heart tire, sleeplessness, and the circulation of unnecessary toxins from a bad condition of the bowels and from improperly selected food all make this complication more liable, its occurrence is, nevertheless, often unpreventable.

The most efficacious preventive pleasures are sleep, rest, the stopping of pain, prevention of exertion, proper food which does not cause flatulence or other indigestion, good, sufficient daily movements of the bowels, the prevention of intestinal distention, and maintenance of a clean, moist surface of the body, produced by such sponging and bathing as the temperature demands.

The disease having developed, the indications for treatment are really few; in fact, the treatment is mostly negative. There is generally but little local pain; the temperature from simple endocarditis alone is not high and the acute symptoms tend to abate.

Local Treatment.—Endocarditis having been diagnosed, especially if there is palpation or pain, an ice bag over the heart is often of considerable value, but not so efficient as in pericarditis. It often tends to quiet the heart, and may be of some value reflexly in slowing the inflammation. If it causes restlessness, however, and does not lessen the pain (which in some instances it may increase), it certainly should be stopped. Children, in whom this complication so frequently occurs, generally do not bear the ice bag well. Sometimes it may be advisable to substitute warm applications, and often a great deal of comfort is derived from them, the patient soon going to sleep. One of the greatest values of either cold or hot applications is diminution of the discomfort from the cardiac disturbance, and the stopping of any pain which may be present. If they do not do this, there is no object in using either cold or heat.

The discomfort from blisters over the heart during the acute stage of endocarditis is greater than any good which they can do. In adults a few small blisters may be used intermittently around the borders of the heart, after the acute symptoms are over, to act reflexly on the heart and possibly aid absorption of inflammatory products. Sometimes improvement seems to follow such treatment; it certainly can do no harm.

During convalescence, the skin over the heart may be painted with iodin, repeated often enough to cause stimulation without injuring the skin; it seems at times to be of value. Various iodin or iodid ointments have been used, but they probably have no more value than the administration of small doses of iodid.

Systemic Treatment.—As this complication most frequently occurs during acute rheumatism, the question arises as to the value or harmfulness of salicylates and alkaline drugs. With our recent better understanding of the action on the heart of pure salicylates (either natural or synthetic saliclic acid, which have been shown to act identically, if equally pure), we must believe that in any ordinary dosage they will injure the heart but rarely. While salicylic acid will not prevent endocarditis, it should he continued, if it is of benefit with regard to the arthritis. The indication for its use depends on its effect on the joints. As it acts at times almost as a specific in rheumatism, it would seem that it should be of value in the endocarditis caused by rheumatism. On the other hand, the endocarditis occurs during the second or third week of acute rheumatism, after the blood has been thoroughly saturated with salicylic acid. Therefore it certainly does not tend to prevent rheumatic endocarditis; hence for this complication alone salicylic acid is not indicated.

ALKALIES

Anything which tends to increase the acidity of the tissues and to diminish the alkalinity of the blood, whether from starvation or outer causes, seems to pro-duce endocardial and myocardial irritation, if not actual inflammation. Therefore in a disease like rheumatism, which seems to be made worse by anything which increases the acidity, alkalies are obviously indicated, and it is probable that an increased alkalinity of the blood tends to prevent endocardial irritation, and may soothe an inflammation already present. Until we have some positive knowledge to the contrary, alkalies should be freely administered during endocarditis, especially during rheumatic endocarditis. Potassium citrate in 2 gm. (30 grain) closes, in wintergreen water, should be given every three to six hours, depending on how readily the urine is made alkaline. This may be given with the salicylic acid treatment, and also when the salicylic acid has been stopped. It may be well, if sodium salicylate is being used, to give also sodium bicarbonate, the sodium bicarbonate often preventing irritation of the stomach from the sodium salicylate, the dose being equal parts of the sodium salicylate and the sodium bicarbonate administered in plenty of water. If some other form of salicylic acid is preferred, novaspirin, which is methylene-citryl-salicylic acid and contains 62 percent of salicylic acid, is perhaps the least irritant to the stomach of the salicylic preparations. This drug is decomposed in the intestine into its component parts, salicylic acid and methylene-citric acid. If this drug is combined with sodium bicarbonate, the disintegration into its component parts would be likely to occur in the stomach.

IRON

It is essential for the welfare of the patient, especially after a long illness before the complication of endocarditis could occur, and in rheumatic fever, in which all meat and meat extractives have been kept from the diet, that small doses of iron should be administered daily. Not only the fever process, but also the salicylic acid tends to prevent the healthy normal growth of red corpuscles. and such patients suffering from rheumatism are often seriously anemic after the aente inflammation has ceased. The iron administered may be 5 drops of the tincture of the chlorid, in lemonade or orangeade, twice in twenty-four hours (and it should be remembered that lemon and orange burn to alkalies in the system and do not act as acids); or 0.1 gm. (1 1/2 grains) of reduced iron in capsule twice in twenty-four hours, or a 3 grain tablet of saccharated ferric oxid (Eisenzucker) twice in twenty-four hours.

OPIUM

As so many times repeated, real pain must be stopped, and morphin, either by the mouth or hypodermically, should be used to the point of stopping such pain. If the patient is a young child, codein sulphate or the deodorized tincture of opium may be used in the dose found sufficient, and either one will act satisfactorily. The dose given should be small but repeated sufficiently often to stop the pain. The dose necessary for the given individual will soon be learned, and that dose may be repeated at such intervals as the condition may require. Sometimes the hypnotic selected, if one is needed, will be sufficient to quiet the cardiac aches or pains.

BROMIDS AND CHLORAL

If there is much restlessness and the circulation is good, that is, if myocarditis is probably not present, the bromids may be of great value, especially in children. The dose should be sufficient to quiet the nervous system. The drug may be discontinued after a few days, if the conditions improve. If the bromid, except in large doses, will not cause sleep, a sufficient dose of chloral should be given. Chloral is one of the most satisfactorily acting drugs which we have to produce sleep and to cause cardiac rest. While it should not be given if there is real cardiac weakness, the good which it does is so much greater than the possible bad effect on the heart, that it should not be forgotten for some newer hypnotic. The worst part of this drug is its taste, and the best way to administer it is to have it in solution in water and the dose given on cracked ice with a little lemon juice to be followed by a good drink of water and a piece of orange pulp for the patient to chew. Ordinarily a bad-tasting drug such as chloral is well administered in effervescing water, but effeverscing waters are generally inadvisable when there is any kind of inflammation of the heart, as they are liable to cause distention of the stomach and pressure on the heart. Some physicians prefer chloralamid as a less disagreeable drug and one which acts almost as efficiently as chloral. As the close of this must be larger than the dose of chloral, it is a question of doubt as to which is the better drug to use. Of the newer hypnotics, veronal=sodium (sodium-diethyl-barbiturate) is among the best. It acts quickly, is less depressant and is a safer salt than most of the other newer hypnotics. It is the readily soluble sodium salt of veronal (diethyl-barbituric acid). When combined with any active drug, sodium seems to make it less toxic and less depressant. The dose of this drug is from 0.2 to 0.3 gm. (3 to 5 grains).

PREVENTION

If the patient is weak, the circulation depressed, the blood pressure low, and the heart rapid, the drug advisable to produce rest and sleep is almost always morphin or some other form of opium. Morphin, with few exceptions, is a cardiac tonic and a cardiac stimulant, unless the dose is much too large. As long as the bowels are daily moved and the food is not given at the time of the full action of the morphin, when digestion might be delayed or interfered with, in most patients the action of this drug during serious illness is entirely for good. The greatest mistake in using morphin for the production of sleep, or for physical and mental rest and comfort when there is not severe pain, is in giving too large a dose. If pain is not severe, or due to inflammatory distention of some undilatable part, to pressure on some nerve, to distention of some tube by a calculus or to some serious injury to the nerves, large doses of morphin are not needed. Small doses will act much more efficiently. It is excessively rare that a hypodermic of one- fourth grain of morphin sulphate is needed, except for the conditions enumerated. It is often a fact that so small a dose as one-eighth grain of morphin or even one-sixth grain will cause sufficient stimulation of a nervous patient, because its primary stimulant effect on the spinal cord is greater than its depressant effect on the brain, to require another dose (one-fourth grain altogether) to give such a patient rest. On the other hand, this patient may many times be quieted by one-tenth grain of morphin sulphate on account of the size of the dose being not sufficient to stimulate the spinal cord. Many a time clinically when one-eighth grain has failed, a dose of one-fourth grain having been apparently necessary, a change to one-tenth grain has proved entirely and perfectly satisfactory.

DIET

As intimated in the preceding paragraph, the diet during endocarditis must be carefully regulated. It must be sufficient, and appropriate for the disease in which the complication occurs, but it must be in such dosage and administered with such frequency as to cause the least possible indigestion. Large amounts of milk are rarely advisable. Too much milk is certainly given, even in rheumatism. While pretty well tolerated by children, it is often badly tolerated as far as digestive symptoms are concerned, by adults. The amount of liquid given should be governed by the amount of urine passed and by the amount of perspiration. The patient should not be overloaded with liquid if he does not need it. Enough carbohydrate must be given.

LAXATIVES

If the bowels are known to be in excellent condition and not loaded with fecal matters, brisk catharsis is not needed simply because endocarditis has developed. If the bowels have been neglected, a small dose of calomel, aided by a compound aloin tablet, is necessary and good treatment. Subsequent movements of the bowels should be daily obtained by vegetable laxatives with occasional enemas, as needed. With all inflammation of the heart and the possibility of myocarditis developing or being actually present, it is not advisable to use salines freely or often.

CARDIAC DRUGS

Whether any drug should be used which acts directly on the heart is often a question for decision. As endocarditis is generally secondary to some acute disease, the patient has become weakened already, and the circulation is not sturdy; therefore such a drug as aconite is probably never indicated. The necessary diminished diet, catharsis, hypnotic, salicylic acid and alkalies all tend to quiet the circulation and diminish any strenuosity of the heart that may be present. Unfortunately, during fever processes, digitalis in ordinary doses rarely slows the heart; and while it might slow the heart if given in large doses, it would also cause too powerful contractions of the ventricles. Digitalis is inadvisable if there is much endocardial inflammation, and especially if there is supposed or presumed to be acute myocardial inflammation. If a patient had already valvular disease from a previous endocarditis, and during this attack insufficiency of the heart was evidenced by pendent edemas, digitalis Should be administered; but it probably should not be given to other patients during the acute period of inflammation.

BATHS

During rheumatism the peripheral blood vessels are generally dilated and the skin perspires profusely. This is caused not only by the rheumatism, but also by the salicylates. The surface of the body should be sponged with cold, lukewarm or hot water, depending on the temperature, especially of the skin. The cold water will reduce the temperature and tone the peripheral blood vessels; the hot water, if the temperature is low and the skin moist and flabby, will cleanse it and also tone the peripheral blood vessels. If the blood vessels are dilated and the perspiration profuse, atropin is indicated, both as a cardiac stimulant and contractor of the blood vessels and as a preventer of too profuse sweating. The dose should be from 1/200 to 1/100 grain for an adult, given two or three times in twenty-four hours, depending on its action and the indications. It should be remembered that atropin is not a sleep-producer; it may stimulate the cerebrum. Therefore at night it might well be combined with a possible necessary hypodermic injection of morphin.

STRYCHNIN

The question of the advisability of strychnin is a constant subject for discussion. Strychnin is overused in the cases of most patients who are seriously ill. In a patient in whom we are trying to cause nervous and muscular rest, strychnin is certainly contraindicated. On the other hand, if the heart is acting sluggishly, the peripheral circulation is imperfect, and atropin is not acting well, it is advisable to give strychnin in a dose not too large and not too frequently repeated. Strychnin should be avoided, if possible, in the evening in order that the patient may sleep. Whether it should be given by the mouth or hypodermically would depend entirely on the seriousness of the condition. Once in six hours is generally often enough for strychnin to be administered unless the dose is very small.

ALCOHOL

It is rarely, if ever, advisable to use alcohol. In certain instances, however, especially in older patients who are accustomed to alcohol, a little whisky administered several times a day may act only for good, both as a food and as a peripheral dilator. But it must be remembered that alcohol is not a cardiac stimulant, and that a large dose will be followed by more cardiac depression. Nitroglycerin may act as well as whisky in the kind of cases mentioned. Caffein stimulation in any form is generally inadvisable during inflammation of the heart.

PROGNOSIS AND CONVALESCENCE

The duration of acute endocarditis varies greatly; it may be two or three weeks, or the inflammation may become subacute and last for several months. Although mild endocarditis rarely causes death of itself, it may develop into an ulcerative endocarditis, and then be serious per se. On the other hand, it may add its last quota of disability to a patient already seriously ill, and death may occur from the combination of disturbances. As soon as all acute symptoms have ceased, rheumatic or otherwise, and the temperature is normal, the amount of food should be increased; the strongly acting drugs should be stopped; the alkalies, especially, should not be given too long, and the salicylates should be given only intermittently, if at all; iron should be continued, massage should be started, and iodid should be administered, best in the form of the sodium iodid, from 0.1 to 0.2 gm. (1 1/2 to 3 grains), twice in twenty-four hours, with the belief that it does some good toward promoting the resorption of the endocardial inflammatory products and can never do any harm. Prolonged bed rest must be continued, visitors must still be proscribed, long conversations must not be allowed, and the return to active mental and physical life must be most deliberate.

No clinician could state the extent to which the valvular inflammation will improve or how much disability of the valves must be permanent. It is even stated by some clinicians that a rest in bed for three months is advisable. While this is of course excessive, certainly, when the future health and ability of the patient are under consideration, and especially when the patient is a child or an adolescent, time is no object compared with the future welfare of the person's heart. It is one of the greatest pleasures of a the clinician to note such a previously inflamed heart gradually diminish in size and the murmurs at the valves affected gradually disappear. Although they may have disappeared while the patient is in bed, he is not safe from the occurrence of a valvular lesion for several months after he is up and about.

While the discussion of hygiene would naturally be confined to the hygiene of the disease of which the endocarditis is a complication, still the hygiene of its most frequent cause, rheumatism, should be referred to. Fresh air and plenty of it, and dry air if possible, is what is needed in rheumatism, and a shut-up, over-heated and especially a damp room will continue rheumatism indefinitely. It is almost as serious for rheumatism as it is for pneumonia. Sunlight and the action of the sun's rays in a rheumatic patient's bedroom are essential, if possibly obtainable.

As so many rheumatic germs are absorbed from diseased or inflamed tonsils or from other parts of the mouth and throat, proper gargling or swashing of the mouth and throat should be continued as much as possible, even during an endocarditis. The prevention of mouth infections will be the prevention of rheumatism and of endocarditis.

MALIGNANT ENDOCARDITIS: ULCERATIVE ENDOCARDITIS

Since we have learned that bacteria are probably at the bottom of almost any endocarditis, the terms suggested under the classification of endocarditis as "mild" and "malignant" really represent a better understanding of this disease. They are not separate entities, and a mild endocarditis may become an ulcerative endocarditis with malignant symptoms. On the other hand, malignant endocarditis may apparently develop de novo. Still, if the cause is carefully sought there will generally be found a source of infection, a septic process somewhere, possibly a gonorrhea, a septic tonsil or even a pyorrhea alveolaris. Septic uterine disturbances have long been known to be a source of this disease. Meningitis, pneumonia, diphtheria, typhoid fever and rarely rheumatism may all cause this severe form of endocarditis.

Ulcerative endocarditis was first described by Kirkes in 1851, was later shown to be a distinctive type of endocarditis by Charcot and Virchow, and finally was thoroughly described by Osler in 1885.

Ulcerative endocarditis was for a long time believed to be inevitably fatal; it is now known that a small proportion of patients with this disease recover. Children occasionally suffer from it, but it is generally a disease of middle adult life. Chorea may bear an apparent causal relation to it in rare instances.

Ulcerative endocarditis may develop on a mild endocarditis, with disintegration of tissue and deep points of erosion, and there may be little pockets of pus or little abscesses in the muscle tissue. If such a process advances far, of course the prognosis is absolutely dire. If the ulcerations, though formed, soon begin to heal, especially in rheumatism, the prognosis may be good, as far as the immediate future is concerned. If the process becomes septic, or if there is a serious septic reason for the endocarditis, the outlook is hopeless. This form of endocarditis is generally accompanied by a bacteremia, and the causative germs may be recovered from the blood. One of the most frequent is the Streptococcus viridans.

DIAGNOSIS

If a more malignant form of endocarditis develops on a mild endocarditis, the diagnosis is generally not difficult. If, without a definite known septic process, malignant endocarditis develops, localized symptoms of heart disturbance and cardiac signs may be very indefinite.

If there is no previous disease with fever, the temperature from this endocarditis is generally intermittent, accompanied by chills, with high rises of temperature, even with a return to normal temperature at times. There may be prostration and profuse sweats. Even without emboli there may be meningeal symptoms: headache, restlessness, delirium, dislike of light and noise, and stupor; even convulsions may occur. The urine generally soon shows albumin; there may be joint pains; the spleen is enlarged and the liver congested. Some definite cardiac symptoms are soon in evidence, with more or less progressive cardiac weakness. Occasionally there are no symptoms other than the cardiac.

Characteristic of this inflammation is the development of ecchymotic spots on the surface of the body, especially on the feet and lower extremities. Sooner or later, in most instances of the severe form of this disease, emboli from the ulcerations in the heart reach the different organs of the body, and of course the symptoms will depend on the place in which the emboli locate. If in the abdomen, there are colicky pains with disturbances, depending on the organs affected; if in the brain, there may be paralysis, more or less complete. In all infaret occurs in one of the organs of the body there must of necessity occur a necrosis of the part and an added focus of infection. If a peripheral artery is plugged, gangrene of the part will generally occur, if the patient lives long enough.

TREATMENT

If pneumonia or gonorrhea is supposed to be the cause of the endocarditis, injections of stock vaccines should perhaps be used. If the form of sepsis is not determinable, streptococcic or staphylococcic vaccines might be administered. It is still a question whether such "shotgun" medication with bacteria is advisable. Patients recover at times from almost anything, and the interpretation of the success of such injection treatment is difficult. Exactly how much harm such injections of unnecessary vaccines can produce in a patient is a question that has not been definitely decided. Theoretically an autogenous vaccine is the only vaccine which should be successful. The vaccine treatment of ulcerative endocarditis was not shown to be very successful by Dr. Frank Billings [Footnote: Billings, Frank: Chronic Infectious Endocarditis, Arch. Int. Med., November, 1909, p. 409.] in his investigation, and more recent treatment of this disease, when caused by the Streptococcus viridons, by antogenous vaccines has confirmed his opinion.

Other treatment of malignant endocarditis includes treatment of the condition which caused it plus treatment of "mild" endocarditis, as previously described, with meeting of all other indications as they occur. As in all septic processes, the nutrition must be pushed to the full extent to which it can be tolerated by the patient, namely, small amounts of a nutritious, varied diet given at three-hour intervals.

Whether milk or any other substance containing lime makes fibrin deposits on the ulcerative surfaces more likely or more profuse, and therefore emboli more liable to occur, is perhaps an undeterminable question. In instances in which hemorrhages so frequently occur, as they do in this form of endocarditis, calcium is theoretically of benefit. Quinin has not been shown to be of value, and salicylic acid is rarely of value unless the cause is rheumatism.

Alcohol has been used in large doses, as it has been so frequently used in all septic processes. If the patient is unable to take nourishment in any amount, small doses of alcohol may be of benefit. It is probably of no other value. It is doubtful whether ammonium carbonate tends to prevent fibrin deposits or clots in the heart, as so long supposed. In fact, whenever the nutrition is low and the patient is likely to have cerebral irritation from acidemia, whenever the kidneys are affected, or whenever a disease may tend to cause irritation of the brain and convulsions, it is doubtful if ammonium carbonate or aromatic spirit of ammonia is ever indicated. Ammonium compounds have been shown to be a cause of cerebral irritation. Salvarsan has not been proved of value.

Intestinal antisepsis may be attained more or less successfully by the administration of yeast or of lactic acid ferments together with suitable diet. The nuclein of yeast may be of some value in promoting a leukocytosis. It has not been shown, however, that the polymorphonuclear leukocyte increase caused by nuclein has made phagocytosis more active.

Malignant endocarditis may prove fatal in a few days, or may continue in a slow subacute process for weeks or even months.

CHRONIC ENDOCARDITIS

It is not easy to decide just whew all acute endocarditis has entirely subsided and a chronic, slow-going inflammation is substituted. It would perhaps be better to consider a slow-going inflammatory process subsequent to acute endocarditis as a subacute endocarditis; and an infective process may persist in the endocardium, especially in the region of the valves, for many weeks or perhaps months, with some fever, occasional chills, gradually increasing valvular lesions and more or less general debility and systemic symptoms. Such a subacute endocarditis may develop insidiously on a previously presumably healed endocardial lesion and cause symptoms which would not be associated with the heart, if an examination were not made. Sometimes such a slow-going inflammatory process will be associated with irregular and intangible chest pains, with some cough or with many symptoms referred to the stomach, so that the stomach may be considered the organ which is at fault. There may be dizziness, headache, feelings of faintness, sleeplessness, progressive debility and a persistent cough, with some bronchial irritation and with occasional expectoration of streaks of blood, which may cause the diagnosis of incipient tuberculosis to be made. The need of a careful general examination must be emphasized again before a decision is made as to what ails the patient, or before cough mixtures are given unnecessarily, quinin is prescribed for supposed malarial chills, or various diets and digestants are recommended for a supposed gastric disturbance.

The term "chronic endocarditis" should be reserved for a slowly developing sclerosis of the vavles. This may occur in a previous rheumatic heart and in a heart which has suffered endocarditis and has valvular lesions, or it may occur from valvular strain or heart strain from various causes; it is typically a part of the arteriosclerotic process of age, and is then mostly manifested at the aortic valve.

ETIOLOGY

Rheumatism is the cause of most instances of cardiac disease which date back to childhood or youth, while arteriosclerosis and chronic infection cause most cardiac diseases in the adult. In the former case it is the mitral valve which is the most frequently affected, while in the latter it is the aortic valve. Any cause which tends to induce arteriosclerosis may be a cause of chronic endocarditis, such as gout, syphilis, chronic nephritis, alcoholism, excessive use of tobacco, excessive muscular labor and hard athletic work. Lead is also another, now rather infrequent, cause. Severe infections may tend to make not only an arteriosclerosis occur early in life, but also a chronic endocarditis. Heart strain may also be a cause of chronic endocarditis, especially at the aortic valve. Forced marches of soldiers, competitive athletic feats, and occupations which call for repeated hard physical strain may all cause aortic valve disease. Tobacco, besides increasing the blood tension and thus perhaps injuring the aortic valve, may weaken the heart muscle and cause disturbance and irritation and perhaps inflammation of the mitral valve.

There is no age which is exempt from valvular disease, but the age determines the valve most liable to be affected. If endocarditis occurs in the fetus, it is the right side of the heart that is affected; in children and during adolescence it is most frequently the mitral valve that is involved; while in the adult or in old age it is the aortic valve that is most liable to become diseased. Statistics have shown that the valves of the left side of the heart are diseased nearly twenty times as frequently as those of the right side of the heart. They also show that the mitral valve is diseased more than one and one-half times as frequently as the aortic valve. Early in life probably the two sexes are equally affected with valvular disease, with perhaps a slight preponderance among females, because of their greater tendency to chorea. Females also show a greater frequency to mitral stenosis than do males. Aortic disease, on the other hand, from the very fact of their strenuous life and occupations, is nearly three times more frequent in men than in women.

PATHOLOGY

If a chronic endocarditis has followed an acute condition, some slight permanent papillomas or warty growths may he left from the healed granulating or ulcerated surfaces. Sometimes these little elevations on the valves become inflamed and then adhere together, or adhere to the wall of the heart, and thus incapacitate a valve. Sometimes these excrescences undergo partial fatty degeneration, or may take on calcareous changes and thus stiffen a valve.

If the chronic inflammation is not superimposed on an acute endocarditis there may be no cell infiltration and therefore no softening, but there is a tendency to develop a fibrillated structure, and a fibroid thickening of the endocardium occurs, especially around the valves. This induration causes contraction and narrowing of the orifices with shortening and thickening of the chordae tendineae, and the valves imperfectly open, or no longer close. Fatty degeneration may occur in the papillary growths with necrotic changes, and this may lead to the formation of atheromatous ulcers which may later become covered with lime deposits, and then a hard calcareous ring may form. Fibrin readily deposits on this calcareous substance and may form a permanent capping, or may slowly disintegrate and allow fragments to fly off into the blood stream and cause more or less serious embolic obstruction. If this chronic endocarditis develops with a general arteriosclerosis, the wine inflammation soon occurs in the aorta, and, following the endarteritis in the aorta, atheromatous deposits may also occur there. Chronic endocarditis of the walls of the heart, not in immediate continuity with endocarditis of the valves, is perhaps not liable to occur, except with myocarditis.

TREATMENT

A subacute or a chronic infective endocarditis should be treated on the same plan as an acute endocarditis, which means rest in bed and whatever medication seems advisable, depending on the supposed cause of the condition.

A chronic endocarditis which is part of a general arteriosclerosis requires no special treatment except that directed toward preventing the advance of the general disease.

CHRONIC DISEASES OF THE VALVES

PATHOLOGIC PHYSIOLOGY

The development of permanent injury to one or more valves of the heart may have been watched by the physician who cares for a patient with acute endocarditis, or it may have been noted early during the progress of arteriosclerosis or other conditions of hypertension. On the other hand, many instances of valvular lesions may be found during a life-insurance examination, or are discovered by the physician making a general physical examination for an indefinable general disturbance or for local symptoms. without the patient ever having known that he had a damaged heart. The previous history of such a patient will generally disclose the pathologic cause or the physical excuse.

As soon as a valve has become injured the heart muscle hypertrophies to force the blood through a narrowed orifice or to evacuate the blood coming into a compartment of the heart from two directions instead of one, as occurs in regurgitation or insufficiency of a valve. The heart muscle becomes hypertrophied, like any other muscle which is compelled to do extra work. Which part or parts of the heart will become most enlarged depends on the particular valvular lesion. In some instances this enlargement is enormous, increasing a heart which normally weighs from 10 to 12 ounces to a weight of 20 or even 25 ounces, and extreme weights of from 40 to 50 ounces and even more are recorded.

As long as the heart remains in this hypertrophied condition, which may be called normal hypertrophy since it is needed for the work which has to be done in overcoming the defect in the valve, there are no symptoms, the pulmonary and systemic circulation is sufficient, and the patient does not know that he is incapacitated. Sooner or later, however, the nutrition of the heart, especially in atheromatous conditions, becomes impaired, and the lack of a proper blood supply to the heart muscle causes myocardial disturbance, either a chronic myocarditis or fatty degeneration. If there is no atheromatous condition of the coronary arteries, and arterial disease is not a cause of the valvular lesion, compensation may be broken by some sudden extra strain put on the heart, either muscular or by some acute sickness or a necessary anesthetic and operation. From any of these causes the muscle again becomes impaired, and the heart, especially the part which is the weakest and has the most work to do relatively to its strength, becomes dilated, compensation is broken, and all of the various circulatory disturbances resulting from an insufficient heart strength develop.

PRECAUTIONS TO BE OBSERVED

As long as compensation is complete, there are no medication and physical treatment necessary for the damaged heart. The patient, however, should be told of his disability, and restrictions in his habits and life should be urged on him. The most important are that all strenuous physical exercise should be interdicted; competitive athletics should be absolutely prohibited; prolonged muscular effort must never be attempted, whether running, rowing, wrestling, bicycle riding, carrying a heavy weight upstairs or overlifting in any form. The patient should be taught that he should never rush upstairs, and that he should never run rapidly for a car or a train or for any other reason; he should not pump up a tire, or repeatedly attempt to crank a refractory engine; even the prolonged tension of steering a car for a long distance is inadvisable. He should be told that after a large meal he is less capacitated for exertion than a man who has not a damaged heart. It is better if he drinks no tea or coffee; it is much better if he absolutely refrains from tobacco and alcohol. Prolonged mental worry, business frets and mental depression are all injurious to his heart. Anything which seriously excites him, whether anger or a stimulating drug, is harmful. Any disease which he may acquire, especially lung disturbances, as pneumonia or even a serious cough, requires that he take better care of himself and be more carefully treated and take more rest in bed than a patient who has not a damaged heart. Anything which raises the blood pressure is of course more serious for his heart than for a perfect heart; therefore drinking large amounts of liquid, even water, is inadvisable. It simply means so much more work for the heart to do. Such patients should rarely be given any drug that causes cardiac debility, and should never take one without advicc. This applies to all the coal-tar drugs, acetylsalicylic acid (aspirin), etc.

One other fact should be impressed on the person with a valvular lesion and compensation, and that is that he has but little, if any, reserve circulatory power. While he is in apparently perfect health, it takes little circulatory strain to push his heart to the point of danger or insufficiency. As nothing keeps this reserve so good or increases it more than rest, he should expect to have a restful day at least once a week, and a good rest of at least two or three weeks once or twice a year.

A patient with these restrictions may live for years with a serious valvular defect and may die of some intercurrent disease which has nothing to do with the circulatory system.

It is easily recognizable that as the majority of acute lesions of the valves occur in children, it is impossible to prevent them from taking more or less strenuous exercise, and this is probably the reason that we have so many serious broken compensations during youth or early adolescence.

As referred to under the subject of myocarditis, many symptoms for which a patient consults his physician are indefinite and intangible, though due to cardiac weakness. If a patient with a damaged heart has a sudden dilatation, of course his symptoms are so serious that the physician is immediately summoned. If, however, he has a slowly developing insufficiency of the heart muscle, his first symptoms are more or less indefinite cardiac pains, slight shortness of breath, slight attacks of palpitation, a dry, tickling, short cough occurring after the least exertion, some digestive disturbances, often sluggishness of the bowels, gastric flatulence, possibly nosebleeds, and sooner or later some edema of the lower extremities at the end of the day.

DECOMPENSATION

To understand the physiology, pathology and the best treatment for broken compensation, it is necessary to study the physics of the circulation under the different conditions. With the mitral valve insufficient, a greater or less amount of blood is regurgitated into the left auricle, which soon becomes dilated. Distention of any hollow muscular organ, if the distention is not to the point of paralysis, means a greater inherent or reflex attempt of that organ to evacuate itself; the muscular tissue begins to grow, and a hypertrophy of the left auricle with the above-named lesion develops. The muscular tissue of the auricle, however, is not sufficient to allow any great hypertrophy. The blood flowing from the pulmonary veins into the left auricle finds this cavity already partly filled with blood regurgitated from the left ventricle. The pulmonary blood, being impeded, tends to flow more slowly, and therefore dams back into the lungs, causing a passive congestion of the lungs. The pulmonary artery thus finds the pressure ahead unusually great, and the right ventricle reflexly learns that it requires a greater force to empty itself than before; in fact, it may not succeed in completely accomplishing this until its distention, by an incomplete evacuation of its contained blood plus the blood coming from the right auricle, has caused the right ventricle also to become hypertrophied. This increased muscular action of the right ventricle relieves the pulmonary congestion, and an increased amount of blood is forced into the left auricle. On account of its hypertrophy, the left auricle is able to send an increased amount of blood into the left ventricle, which in turn becomes hypertrophied and sends enough blood into the aorta to satisfy the requirements of the systemic circulation in spite of the leakage through the mitral valve.

As long as this compensation continues, there are no symptoms. If any dilatation occurs from disease, degeneration or from increased work put on the heart (and it is readily seen how delicate this equilibrium is), signs of broken compensation begin to occur. The left ventricle with its enormous strain is perhaps the first part to dilate, thus enlarging the opening of the defective mitral valve. The left auricle is then unable to cope with the increased amount of regurgitant blood, and there is in consequence congestion in the lungs, and the right ventricle finds the pressure ahead in the lungs greater than it can well overcome. The right ventricle, in its turn being overworked, becomes dilated, and as a result of the inability of the right ventricle to evacuate its contents perfectly, the right auricle is unable to force its venous blood into the right ventricle, and there is then a damming back and sluggish circulation in the superior and inferior venae cavae. The results of these circulatory deficiencies are, in the first place, congestion of the lungs and dyspnea; in the second place, with the impaired force of the left ventricle making the arterial circulation imperfect, and with the impaired return of venous blood to the right auricle making the venous circulation sluggish, passive congestions of various organs occur and are evidenced in headache and venous congestion of the eyes and throat, with perhaps cerebral irritability, sleeplessness, and inability to do good mental work. The sluggish return of the blood in the inferior vena cava causes primarily a sluggish portal circulation with a passive congestion and enlargement of the liver. This causes imperfect bile secretion and an imperfect antidotal action to the various toxins of the body or to any alkaloidal drugs or poisons ingested. This congestion of the liver causes a damming back of the blood in the various veins of the portal system, which causes congestion of the stomach and of the mucous membrane of the bowels, and an imperfect secretion of the digestive fluids of these structures. There is also congestion of the spleen. The imperfect return of the blood through the inferior vena cava also interferes with the return of the blood through the renal veins, and more or less renal congestion occurs, with a concentrated urine and perhaps an albuminuria as the result. The same sluggish flow of the inferior vena cava blood, plus the imperfect tone of the systemic arterial system, means that the circulation at the distal portions of the body—the feet and the legs—is imperfect when the patient is up and about, with the result of causing pendant edemas, which disappear at night when the patient is at rest and the heart more easily accomplishes its work.

The physical signs of such a heart, the increased valvular murmur or murmurs, its irregular action, possibly intermittence or irregular contractions of different parts of the heart, causing diocrotic or intermittent pulse with a lowered blood pressure, are all signs readily found. The quickened respiration is Nature's method of aiding the return circulation in the veins by increasing the negative pressure in the chest. The increased number of pillows the patient requires at night is to aid Nature's need to have a better venous return circulation in the vital centers at the base of the brain.

The dry, troublesome, tickling cough is generally due to a congestion of the blood vessels at the base of the tongue, in the lingual tonsil region, or possibly in the larynx. Later the passive congestion of the lungs may be sufficient to cause a bronchitis, with cough and expectoration.

Sometimes, as indicative of primary cardiac distress, these patients have sharp pains through the heart. Such pains are the exception rather than the rule, and are more likely to occur in chronic myocarditis or in coronary disease: in other words, in true angina pectoris.

If there is considerable venous congestion there may be more or less frequent recurrent venous hemorrhages. This frequently is an epistaxis, or a bleeding from hemorrhoids, or in women profuse menstruation or a metrorrhagia.

It is perfectly understandable from the physics of the condition of broken compensation that anything which improves the tone of the heart and makes it again compensatory removes all of these many disabilities, congestions and subacute inflammations. If, however, these passive congestions are long continued, some organs soon become chronically degenerated. This is especially true of the liver and kidneys.

PHYSICS OF MITRAL STENOSIS

Mitral stenosis, though less common than mitral regurgitation, is a frequent form of disease of the valves, especially in women. Often this condition is associated with regurgitation; but in a simple mitral stenosis the greatest hypertrophy is of necessity in the right ventricle. The left auricle finds it difficult to empty all of its blood into the left ventricle during the ordinary diastole of the heart. This auricle then somewhat hypertrophies, but is unable to prevent more or less damming back of the blood into the lungs through the pulmonary veins. This causes passive congestion of the lungs, and the right ventricle finds that it must labor to overcome the increased resistance in the pulmonary artery, and hypertrophies to overcome this increased amount of work. When this condition has become perfected, compensation is established and the circulation is apparently normal. Nature causes these hearts, when they are disturbed or excited, to pulsate slowly, causing the diastole to be longer than in a heart with mitral regurgitation. This allows more blood to enter the left ventricle, and the left ventricle, acting perfectly on the blood which it receives, causes a good systolic pressure in the aorta and the systemic arteries. The left ventricle in this condition does not become hypertrophied. If the heart does act rapidly and the left ventricle contracts on an insufficient amount of blood, the peripheral pulse is necessarily small and the arterial tension is diminished. Very constant in this condition, and of course noticeable whenever there is pulmonary congestion, is the sharp, accentuated closure of the pulmonary valve. The lungs on the least exertion are always a little overfilled with blood. The pulmonary circulation is always working at a little disadvantage.

The first symptoms of lack of compensation with the lesion of mitral stenosis are lung symptoms—dyspnea, cough, bronchitis, slight cyanosis, sometimes blood streaks in the expectorated mucus and froth, and, if the congestion is considerable, some edema of the posterior part of the lungs, if the patient is in bed. Sooner or later during this failing compensation the right ventricle becomes dilated, and the symptoms of cardiac insufficiency and venous congestion occur, as described above with mitral insufficiency.

Again, as in mitral insufficiency, if compensation is restored in mitral stenosis, these symptoms are improved. These patients, however, are never quite free from dyspnea on exertion. Any inflammation of the lungs, even a severe bronchitis, is more or less serious for the patients and their hearts. The mucous membrane of their bronchial tubes and air vesicles is always hyperemic, and it takes little more congestion to all but close up some of the passages. and dyspnea or asthma, or suffocating, difficult cough is the consequence.

PHYSICS OF AORTIC LESIONS

Next in frequency to mitral insufficiency is aortic insufficiency, which occurs most frequently in men. The cavity of the heart that is most affected by this lesion is the left ventricle, which receives blood both from the left auricle, and regurgitantly from the aorta. This part of the heart, being the strongest muscular portion, is the part most adapted to hypertrophy, and the hypertrophy with this lesion is often enormous. For a long time this large muscular section of the heart can overcome all difficulties of the aortic insufficiency. The pulse, however, will always show the quickly lost arterial pressure of every beat on account of the aorta losing its pressure through the regurgitant flow of blood. Sooner or later, from the impaired aortic tension causing a diminished or imperfect flow of blood through the coronary arteries, impaired nutrition of the heart muscle occurs. In other words, an intestinal or chronic myocarditis or fibrosis develops, with perhaps later a fatty degeneration. When this condition occurs, of course, the repair of the heart is impossible.

This form of valvular lesion is the one that is most likely to cause sudden death. In aortic regurgitation Nature causes the heart to beat rapidly. Such a heart must never beat slowly, as the longer the diastole prevails the more blood will regurgitate into the left ventricle, and death may occur from sudden anemia of the base of the brain. Such a heart may, of course, receive a sudden strain, or the left ventricle may dilate, and yet serious myocarditis or fatty degeneration may not have occurred.

The signs of lack of compensation are generally cardiac distress, rapid heart, insufficiency of the systolic force of the left ventricle, and therefore impaired peripheral circulation, a sluggish return circulation, pendent edemas, and soon, with the left auricle finding the left ventricle. insufficiently emptied, the damming back of the blood is in broken compensation with the mitral lesions.

AORTIC STENOSIS

Aortic narrowing or stenosis is a frequent occurrence in the aged and in arteriosclerosis when the aorta is involved. It is not a frequent single lesion in the young. If it occurs in children or young adults, it is likely to be combined with aortic regurgitation, meaning that the valve hay been seriously injured by an endocarditis.

The first effect of this narrowing is to cause hypertrophy of the left ventricle, and as long as this ventricle is able to force the blood through the narrowed opening at the aortic valve, the general circulation is perfect. Nature again steps in to cause such a heart to heat deliberately, allowing time for the contracting ventricle to force the blood through the narrowed orifice. The blood pressure may be sufficient, or even increased if arteriosclerosis is present, although the rise of the sphygmograph tracing is not so high as normal. If the pressure in the aorta is sufficient from the amount of blood forced into it, the coronary arteries receive enough blood to keep up the nutrition of the heart muscle. Sooner or later, however, the left ventricle will become weakened, especially when there is arteriosclerosis or other hypertension, and chronic endocarditis and fatty degeneration result. If the left ventricle becomes sufficiently weakened or dilated, the same damming back of the blood through the lungs and right heart occurs, and more or less serious signs of broken compensation develop. The main danger, however, with a heart with this lesion, occurring coincidently with arteriosclerosis, is a progressive chronic myocarditis.

OTHER LESIONS

Tricuspid insufficiency, except as rarely found in the fetus, is generally due to a relative insufficiency rather than to an actual disease of the tricuspid valve. In other words, if the right ventricle dilates the valve may be insufficient. Tricuspid stenosis, pulmonary stenosis and pulmonary insufficiency are rare, and are probably nearly always congenital.

The diagnosis as to whether the murmurs heard in the heart are hemic, functional, accidental, or indicative of valvular lesions would be without the scope of this book. It is always presumed that a correct diagnosis has been made, or at least a presumptively correct diagnosis. Frequently more than one murmur and more than one lesion in a heart are present. Often one murmur denotes a permanent lesion, and another may be one that will become corrected when compensation is improved.

SYMPTOMATOLOGY AND TREATMENT OF CHRONIC VALVULAR LESIONS

Before discussing the treatment of broken compensation in general, it may be well to describe briefly the differences in the symptoms and treatment of the various valvular lesions.

MITRAL STENOSIS: MITRAL NARROWING

This particular valvular defect occurs more frequently in women than in men, and between the ages of 10 and 30, and is generally the result of rheumatic endocarditis or chorea, perhaps 60 percent of mitral stenosis having this origin. Other causes are various infections or chronic disease, such as nephritis. Of course, like any valvular lesion, it may be associated with other lesions, and sooner or later in many instances, when the left ventricle becomes dilated or weakened, mitral insufficiency also occurs.

It has sometimes seemed that high blood pressure has caused the left ventricle to act with such force as to irritate this mitral valve, and later develop from such irritation a sclerosis or narrowing, and stenosis occurs. It has been suggested that, though lime may be of advantage in heart weakness, as will be stated later, if the blood is overfull of calcium ions the valvular irritations may more readily have deposits of calcium, in other words, become calcareous, and therefore cause more obstruction. It is quite likely, however, that this sort of deposit is only a piece of the general calcification of tissue in arteriosclerosis and old age, and could not be caused by the administration of calcium to a younger patient, and might then occur in older patients even if substances containing much calcium were kept out of the dict. Calcium metabolisim in arteriosclerosis and in softening of the bones is not well understood.

Patients with this lesion are seriously handicapped when any congestion of the lungs occurs, such as pneumonia, pleurisy, or even bronchitis. Asthma is especially serious in these cases, and these patients rarely live to old age.

The pulse is generally slow, unless broken compensation occurs; dyspnea on exertion is a prominent symptom; the increased secretion of mucus in the bronchial tubes and throat is often troublesome, and there is liable to be considerable cough. If these patients have an acute heart attack, a feeling of suffocation is their worst symptom and the dyspnea may be great, although there may be no tachycardia, these hearts often acting slowly even when there is serious discomfort. When compensation fails, there is an occurrence of all the usual symptoms, as previously described.

The distinctive diagnostic physical sign of this lesion is the diastolic and perhaps presystolic murmur heard over the left ventricle, accentuated at the apex and transmitted some distance to the left of the heart. There is also an accentuated pulmonary closure. To palpation this lesion often gives a characteristic presystolic thrill at and around the apex.

The first symptoms of weakening of the compensation are irregularity in the beat and venous congestion of the head and face, causing bluing of the lips, often nosebleed, and sometimes hemoptysis and insomnia. Later the usual series of disturbances from dilatation of the right ventricle occurs. As previously stated, with the absence of good coronary circulation and the consequent impaired nutrition, the left ventricle may also dilate and the mitral valve may become insufficient. Sudden death from heart failure may occur with this lesion more frequently than with mitral insufficiency but less frequently than with aortic insufficiency.

A particularly dangerous period for women with this lesion is when the blood pressure rises after the menopause and the patients become full-blooded and begin to put on weight. Also, these patients always suffer more or less from cold extremities. In most cases they sleep best and with least disturbance with the head higher than one pillow.

Besides the usual treatment for broken compensation in patients with this lesion, digitalis is of the greatest value, and the slowing of the heart by it, allowing the left ventricle to be more completely filled with the blood coming through the narrowed mitral opening during the diastole, is the object desired. This drug acts similarly on both the right and left ventricles, and though there is no real occasion for stimulation of the left ventricle, and it is the right ventricle that is in trouble, dilated and failing, still a greater force of left ventricle contraction helps the peripheral circulation. The action on the right ventricle contributes greatly to the relief of the patient by sending the blood through the lungs and into the left auricle more forcibly. and the left ventricle receives an increased amount of blood, the congestion in the lungs is relieved, and the dyspnea improves. Perhaps there is no class of cardiac diseases in which more frequent striking relief can be obtained than in these cases of mitral stenosis.

If the congestion of the lungs is very great, and death seems imminent from cardiac paralysis, if cyanosis is serious, and bloody. frothy mucus is being expectorated, venesection and an intramuscular injection of aseptic ergot may be indicated. Digitalis should also be given, hypodermically perhaps, but its action would be too late if it was not aided by other more quickly acting drugs. The physician may often save life by such radical measures.

MITRAL INSUFFICIENCY: MITRAL REGURGITATION

This is the most frequent form of valvular disease of the heart, and is due to a shortening or thickening of the valves, or to some adhesion which does not permit the valve, to close properly, and the blood consequently regurgitates from the left ventricle into the left auricle during the contraction of the ventricle. Such regurgitation may occur without valvular disease if for any reason the left ventricle becomes dilated sufficiently to cause the valve to be insufficient. Such a dilatation can generally be cured by rest and treatment. As with mitral stenosis, the most frequent causes are rheumatism and chorea, with the occasional other causes as previously enumerated.

The characteristic murmur of this lesion is a systolic blow, accentuated at the apex, transmitted to the left of the thorax, generally heard in the back, near the lower end of the scapula, and transmitted upward over the precordia.

Of all cardiac lesions, this is the safest one to have. Sudden death is unusual, the compensation of the heart seems to be most readily maintained, and the patient is not so greatly dangered by overexertion or by inflammations in the lungs. As in mitral stenosis, any increase in blood pressure—whether the normal increase after the age of 40, any continued earlier high tension, or increase from occupation or exercise—is serious as causing the left ventricle to act more strenuously, so that more blood is forced back into the left auricle, the lungs become congested, and the right ventricle, sooner or later, becomes incompetent.

When compensation fails with these patients, the first sign is pendent edema of the feet, ankles and legs; subsequently, if there is progressive failure of compensation, the usual symptoms occur.

The treatment is principally rest and digitalis, and the recovery of compensation is often almost phenomenal. Patients with this lesion are likely to be children and young adults, and the heart muscle readily responds as a rule to the treatment inaugurated. Later, in these patients, or if the lesion occurs in older patients, the return to compensation does not occur so readily. If the condition is developed from a myocarditis or from fatty degeneration of the heart, it may be impossible to cause the left ventricle to improve so much as to overcome this relative dilatation or relative insufficiency of the valve. If the dilatation of the left ventricle is due to some poisoning such as nicotin, with proper treatment— stopping the use of tobacco, administration of digitalis, and rest— the heart muscle will generally recover and the valve again properly close.

AORTIC STENOSIS: AORTIC OBSTRUCTION

Valvular disease at the aortic orifice is much less common than at the mitral orifice, and while stenosis or obstruction is less common from rheumatism or acute inflammatory endocarditis than is insufficiency of this valve, a narrowing or at least the clinical sign of narrowing, denoted by a systolic blow at the base of the heart over the aortic opening, is in arteriosclerosis and old age of frequent occurrence. If such narrowing occurs without aortic insufficiency at the age at which it usually occurs, it may not seriously affect the heart. It may follow acute endocarditis, but it most frequently follows chronic endocarditis or atheroma, in which the aortic valves become thickened and more or less rigid; this condition most frequently occurs in men.

Anything that tends to increase arterial tension, as tobacco, lead or hard work, or anything that tends to cause arterial disease, as alcohol or syphilis, is often the cause of this lesion.

At times the edges of the valves may grow together from ulcerative inflammation, and the lumen thus be diminished in size; or projecting vegetations may interfere with the opening of the valve and with the flow of blood. With such narrowing the left ventricle more or less rapidly hypertrophies to overcome its increased work.

The murmur caused by this lesion is a systolic one, either accentuated in the second intercostal space at the right of the sternum, or perhaps heard loudest just to the left of the sternum in this region. The murmur is also transmitted up the arteries into the neck, and may at times be heard in the subclavian arteries. It may also be transmitted downward over the heart. The pulse is slow, the apex of the rise of the sphymographic arterial tracing is more or less sustained and rounded, and the rise is much less than normal.

If this lesion occurs in old age, there is general arterial disease present, and the tension and compressibility of the arteries vary, depending on how much they are hardened. The disturbed circulation is evidenced by imperfect peripheral circulation and capillary sluggishly, with at times pendent edema of the feet and ankles, but, perhaps, little congestion of the lungs. The left ventricle being sufficient, there is no damming back through the left auricle to the lungs. The left ventricle may, however, become weakened, either by some sudden strain or by a chronic myocarditis, and relative insufficiency of the mitral valve may occur. The subsequent symptoms are typically those of loss of compensation.

This lesion may allow a patient to live for years, provided no other serious disturbance of the heart occurs, such as myocarditis or coronary disease; but sooner or later, with the failing force of the blood flow and the lessened aortic pressure, slight attacks of anemia of the brain occur, causing syncope or fainting. Also, sooner or later these patients have little cardiac pains. They begin to "sense" their hearts. There may not be actual anginas, but a little feeling of discomfort, with perhaps pains shooting up into the neck, or a feeling of pressure under the sternum. Little excitements or overexertions are likely to make the heart attempt to contract more rapidly than it is able to drive the blood through the narrowed orifice, and this alone causes cardiac discomfort and the feeling of cardiac oppression.

It is essential, then, that these patients should not hasten and should not become excited; and any drug or stimulant which would cause cardiac excitement is bad for them. On the other hand, these are the very patients in whom, sometimes, alcohol in small doses may be advisable, especially if the patient is old; and a dose of alcohol used medicinally when an attack of cardiac disturbance is present is good treatment. The quick dilatation is valuable. Nitroglycerin will also do good work in these cases, and with high blood tension may be the only safe drug for the patient to have on hand. As soon as his attack occurs, with or without real angina pectoris, let him dissolve in his mouth a nitroglycerin tablet. If he feels faint, he will feel better the moment he lies down, and in this instance he may be improved by a cup of coffee, or a dose of caffein or camphor.

If the left ventricle becomes still weaker and shows signs of serious weakness, or if there is actual dilatation, the question of whether or not digitalis should be used is a subject for careful decision. The left ventricle should not be forced to act too sturdily against this aortic resistance. Consequently the dose of digitalis must be small. On the other hand, it frequently happens, especially in old age, that myocarditis or fatty degeneration has already occurred before this cardiac weakness develops in the presence of aortic narrowing, and digitalis may not be indicated at all. We cannot tell how far degeneration may have gone, however, and small doses of digitalis used tentatively and carefully, perhaps 5 drops of an active tincture two or three times a day, and then the drug carefully increased to a little larger dose to see whether improvement takes place, is the only way to ascertain whether or not digitalis can be used with advantage. If it increases the cardiac pain and distress, it should not be used. Strychnin is then the drug relied on, with such other general medication as is needed, combined with the coincident administration of nitroglycerin, which may also be given in conjunction with digitalis, if deemed advisable. Generally, however, if a heart with aortic stenosis needs stimulation, the blood pressure is generally none too high, although there may be arteriosclerosis present. Therefore when nitroglycerin is indicated to lower blood pressure, digitalis is not usually indicated; when digitalis is indicated to aid the heart, nitroglycerin is generally not indicated. These patients must have high blood pressure to sustain perfect circulation at the base of the brain.

Patients who have this lesion should not use tobacco in large amounts, or sometimes even small amounts, as tobacco raises the blood pressure and thus puts more work on the left ventricle; in the second place, if the left ventricle is failing, much tobacco may hasten its debility. On the other hand, with a failing left ventricle and a long previous use of tobacco, it is no time to prohibit its use absolutely. A failing heart and the sudden stoppage of tobacco may prove a serious combination.

AORTIC INSUFFICIENCY: AORTIC REGURGITATION

This lesion, though not so common as the mitral lesion, is of not infrequent occurrence in children and young adults as a sequence of acute rheumatic endocarditis. If it occurs later in life it generally is associated with aortic narrowing, and is a part of the general endarteritis and perhaps atheroma of the aorta. Sometimes it is caused by strenuous exertion apparently rupturing the valve.

This form of valvular disease frequently ends in sudden death. On the other hand, it is astonishing how active a person may be with this really terrible cardiac defect. This lesion, from the frequent overdistention of the left ventricle, is one which often causes pain. While the left ventricle enlarges enormously to overcome the extra distention due to the blood entering the ventricle from both directions, the muscle sooner or later becomes degenerated from poor coronary circulation. Unless the left ventricle can do its work well enough to maintain an adequate pressure of blood in the aorta, the coronary circulation is insufficient, and chronic myocarditis is the result. If the left ventricle has maintained this pressure for a long time, edemas are not common unless the cardiac weakness is serious and generally permanently serious: that is, slight weakness, in this lesion, does not give edemas as does slight loss of compensation in mitral disease, and unless the weakness of the ventricle is serious, the lungs are not much affected.

The physical sign of this lesion is the diastolic murmur, which is loudest of the base of the heart, is accentuated over the aortic orifice, and is transmitted up into the neck and the subclavians, and down over the heart and down the sternum with marked pulsation, of the arteries (Corrigan pulse) and often of some of the peripheral veins, notably of the arms and throat.

If the left ventricle becomes dilated the mitral valve may become insufficient, when the usual lung symptoms occur, with hypertrophy of the right ventricle; and if it fails, the usual venous symptoms of loss of compensation follow. This lesion not infrequently causes epistaxis, hemoptysis and hematemesis.

Digitalis is always of value in these cases, but it should not be pushed. If a heart is slowed too much, the regurgitation into the left ventricle is increased. Therefore such hearts should not be slowed to less than eighty beats per minute, or sudden anemia of the brain and sudden death may occur. These patients must not do hard work.

TRICUSPID INSUFFICIENCY

This rarely, if ever, occurs alone; it is generally a sequence of other valvular defects, and represents an overworked, dilated right ventricle. It may, however, occur from lesions of the lungs which impede the blood flow through them. Such are fibroid changes in the lungs, emphysema, prolonged chronic bronchitis, the last stages of pulmonary tuberculosis, old neglected pleurisies with cirrhosis or fibrosis of the lung, and repeated attacks of asthma—anything, whether valvular defect or pulmonary circulatory disturbance, which increases the pressure ahead and the work of this ventricle.

The symptoms are those of loss of compensation as described under other valvular lesions. There may be jugular pulsation, especially evident in the external jugular on the left side. The liver enlarges and may pulsate. There are edemas, dropsies, ascites and perhaps hemorrhages. The heart is enlarged and there is a soft systolic blow heard at the lower end of the sternum. The dyspnea is sometimes very great, and cyanosis may be present, especially during paroxysms of coughing.

This lesion of the heart is always benefited by digitalis, but the continuance of the improvement and its amount depend, of course, on the cause of the dilatation of the ventricle. Strychnin is often of advantage. These patients should rarely receive vasodilators, and hot baths, overheating, overloading the stomach and vigorous purging should never be allowed. Sometimes improvement will not take place until ascitic or pleuritic fluid, if present, has been removed.

TRICUSPID STENOSIS: TRICUSPID OBSTRUCTION

This is rare and probably always congenital, and is supposed to be due to an inflammation of the endocardium during intra-uterine life. In early childhood it is possible that it may be associated with left-side endocarditis.

A special treatment of the heart, if any is needed, would probably not be indicated unless there was associated tricuspid insufficiency, when digitalis might be used.

PULMONARY INSUFFICIENCY: PULMONARY REGURGITATION

If this rare condition occurs, it is probably congenital. A distinctive murmur of this insufficiency would be diastolic and accentuated in the second intercostal space on the left of the sternum. It should be remembered that aortic murmurs are often more plainly heard at the left of the sternum. Sooner or later, if this lesion is actually present, the right ventricle dilates and cyanosis and dyspnea occur. Digitalis would therefore be indicated.

PULMONARY STENOSIS: PULMONARY OBSTRUCTION

If stenosis is actually present in this location, the lesion is probably congenital. It might occur after a serious acute infectious endocarditis, but then it would be associated with other lesions of the heart. It has been found to be associated with such congenital lesions of the heart as an open foramen ovale or foramen Botalli, or with an imperfect ventricular septum, and perhaps with tricuspid stenosis—in short, a cardiac congenital defect. The right ventricle becomes hypertrophied, if the child lives to overcome the obstruction.

The physical sign is a systolic blow at the second intercostal space on the left; but as just stated, such a murmur must surely be dissociated from an aortic murmur if found to develop after babyhood, and it should also be diagnosed from the frequently occurring hemic, basic and systolic murmurs; that is, if signs of pulmonary lesions are not heard soon after birth or in early babyhood, the diagnosis of pulmonary defects can be made only by exclusion.

Unless the right ventricle is found later to be in trouble, there is no treatment for this condition. If the right ventricle dilates, digitalis may be of benefit.

ACUTE CARDIAC SYMPTOMS: ACUTE HEART ATTACK

It is not proposed here to describe the condition of sudden cardiac failure, or acute dilatation during disease, or after a severe heart strain, but to describe the terrible cardiac agony which occurs, sometimes repeatedly, with many patients who have valvular lesions. These patients may not have the symptoms of loss of compensation. Probably some one or more chambers of the heart become overdistended and act irregularly, or the blood is suddenly dammed up in the lungs, with the oppression and dyspnea caused by such passive congestion, or perhaps it is the right ventricle that is suddenly in serious trouble.

A physician receives an emergency call, and knows, if it is not a patient who has hysteria, that it is his duty to see the patient immediately. The friends of the patient all anxiously await the physician's arrival; front doors are often wide open, and the servants and the whole household are in a great state of excitement and anxiety. The position in which the patient will be found is that which he has learned gives him the greatest comfort. If the physician knows his patient, he will know how he will find him. He may lie sitting up in bed; he may be standing, leaning over a chair; he may be sitting in a chair leaning over a table or leaning over the back of another chair; but he is using every auxiliary muscle he possesses to respire. He is generally bathed in cold perspiration; the extremities are often icy cold; he calls for air, and to stop fanning all in one breath; he wishes the perspiration wiped off his brow, and nearly goes frantic while it is being done; there is agony depicted on his face; his eyes stare; his expirations are often groaning. Sometimes there is even incontinence of urine and feces, often hiccup or short coughs, perhaps vomiting, and possibly sharp pangs of pain in the cardiac region. A patient with these symptoms may die at any moment, and the wonder is that so many times one lives through these paroxysms.

The patient can hardly be questioned, can certainly not be carefully examined; and herein lies the advantage of the family physician who knows the patient and his heart, and in whom the patient has confidence.

In fact, this confidence which such a patient has in the physician who has more or less frequently aided him in weathering these terrible attacks is alone the greatest boon the patient can have.

MANAGEMENT

The immediate conditions to meet are the rapid fluttering heart, the nervous excitation and cardiac anxiety, and perhaps the most important of all, the vasomotor spasm that is often so pronounced. Physically we have, then, a heart with leaking or constricted valves; in either case more blood is entering the chambers of the heart than can be expelled in one contraction, while the peripheral resistance due to the spasm of the blood vessels, because of fear, becomes greater every minute and tends still more to interfere with the peripheral circulation and the complete emptying of the heart of its surplus blood. Owing to the well known stimulus to distention of hollow muscular organs, the heart contracts faster and faster.

Soon, by some disarrangement of the inhibitory apparatus, the pneumogastric nerves, the heart loses its governor, and the beats increase to even 150 a minute, with irregular contractions, the blood being sent through the arteries with irregular force, as evidenced by the varying volume of the pulse. At this time, with or without cardiac pain, which upsets the rhythm of the heart, the patient becomes frightened at the feeling of impending demise, and the cerebral reflexes begin to add to the cardiac difficulty. The breathing becomes nervously rapid, besides that which is due to the rapid heart. The chill of fear is added to the already contracted peripheral vessels, and the surface of the body becomes cold, the extremities sometimes intensely so. Next it seems as if the strongly contracted arterioles begin actually to prevent some of the peripheral circulation, the blood is piled up in the large arteries, and the venous circulation becomes more and more sluggish, while the lips, finger nails and forehead become cyanotic. Respiration becomes more rapid and deep; the inspiration being as strong as possible with every auxiliary muscle taking part, thus making the negative pressure in the chest aid in bringing the blood back through the veins. Part of the extra respiratory stimulus comes from the imperfectly aerated blood reaching the respiratory center.

Two factors may normally, without treatment, stop these paroxysms, and the "bad heart turn" may be cured spontaneously. The first of these is self-control. If the patient does not lose his head, by an effort of the will he saves himself from becoming nervous or frightened and therefore escapes the result of mental excitement; the increased peripheral blood pressure from fear does not occur, and in a shorter or longer time the heart quiets down. The physician recognizes this power, and gives his patient immediate assurance that he will soon be all right; the patient who knows his physician immediately feels this assurance and is quickly improved.

The second factor in spontaneous cure of the heart attack is relaxation. The exhaustion from the respiratory muscular efforts, together with the drowsy condition caused by the cerebral hyperemia and from the imperfectly aerated blood, causes finally a dulling of the mental acuity, and the nervous excitement abates, which, with the exhaustion, gives a relaxation of peripheral arterioles: the resistance to the flow of the blood is removed, the surface of the body becomes warm, the heart quiets down by the equalization of the circulation, and the paroxysm is over.

DRUGS

The part the nervous system plays in this paroxysm is shown by the good result obtained from injections of morphin, even when there is no pain; hence the action of morphin is directly in line with the natural resolution of the symptoms: it quiets the nervous system, causes drowsiness, relaxes spasm, and thus causes increased peripheral circulation; many times this is the only treatment necessary.

During these heart attacks it is more than useless to administer any drug by the stomach, as in this condition there will be no absorption, even if there is no vomiting.

While morphin is generally indicated, as just suggested, a very large dose should not be given, lest the activity of the respiratory center be impaired (it is already in trouble), and undoubtedly death may easily be caused by an overaction of morphin during these heart attacks. The addition of atropin to the morphin will prevent depression from the morphin. Also, atropin sometimes quiets cardiac pain, but it will not steady the heart, may irritate it, and will increase vasomotor tension, although peripheral nerve irritation may be diminished. Hence a fair dose of morphin hypodermicaly with a small dose of atropin, if respiratory depression is feared, is a physiologic method of bettering the condition. In this kind of heart attack a drug which often acts well is nitroglycerin. It may be given hypodermically in a dose of from 1/200 to 1/100 grain, or a tablet may be dissolved on the tongue, and the dose be repeated once or twice at fifteen-minute intervals, until there is throbbing in the forehead, which shows that a sufficient amount of the drug has been administered. This headache will generally not last long. In the meantime the peripheral blood vessels are relaxed, the surface of the body becomes warm, the heart quiets, and the attack is over. To hasten the action of nitroglycerin (that is, to equalize the circulation) a hot foot-bath is often valuable. Amyl nitrite may be inhaled with the same object in view, but the action is very intense, the prostration often severe, and unless there is angina pectoris, nitroglycerin is much better.

The symptoms of a heart attack may not be quite those described above; they may be those of sudden dilatation or semiparalysis of the heart, in which the prostration is intense and the patient is unable to sit up, although he may be leaning against several pillows. There is dyspnea, but the patient cannot aid respiration with the auxiliary muscles by holding the arms and shoulders tense or obtaining support from the aruls; in fact, the arms are almost strengthless. The surface of the body may be warm, and the arms may be warm except the hands; the feet, ankles and legs may be cold. There is generally more or less cyanosis, although the face may be pale. The finger nails often show venous stasis. In these cases the blood pressure is subnormal, the pulse may be hardly perceptible, and there is none of the tension of the body from fear. The patient may be fearful, but lie is completely collapsed. Such an attack may occur suddenly in a heart that is perfectly compensating, or it may accompany general edemas and dropsies.

If the emergency is excessively urgent, the lungs filling up with blood, moist rales beginning to occur, and frothy and blood-tinged sputum being coughed up, venesection may be indicated; combined with proper hypodermic medication it may save life, and does at times. In fact, a patient who shows every sign of fatal cardiac collapse may be saved. (one of the best drugs to administer to such patient is an aseptic ergot, injected intramuscularly.) The drug of all drugs for future action (as it will not act immediately) is digitalis, given hypodermically.

Whether digitalis shall be given at all, or how large the dose shall be depends on whether or not the patient has been taking digitalis in large quantities.

He may already be overpowered with digitalis. In that case it would be contraindicated.

Stroplianthin, especially when given intravenously, has been found to be a quickly acting circulatory stimulant. The dose of strophanthin, Merck, ranges from 1/500 to l/200 grain. The intravenous dose of strophanthin, Thoms, is about 1/130 grain. It should not be repeated within a day or two, if at all. Ampules of strophanthin in solution for intravenous use are now available.

Atropin in a dose of 1/150 grain, and strychnin in a dose of 1/40 or 1/30 grain are valuable aids in stimulating the circulation under these conditions. The atropin should not be repeated. The strychnin may be repeated in three, four or five hours, depending on the size of the previous close.

Of all quickly acting stimulants, none is better than camphor in saturated solution in sterile oil as may be obtained in ampules. Alcohol is absolutely contraindicated in the latter condition. In the former kind of heart attack, vasodilation from a large close of whisky or brandy may be of value. The dose should be large to cause immediate increased peripheral circulation, dilation, and even a little stupefaction of the central nervous system, and it may be effectual in a way not dissimilar to the action of morphiti.

TREATMENT OF BROKEN COMPENSATION

The consideration of this subject will include the following topics:

A. Hygiene.

B. Diet.

C. Elimination.

D. Physical measures.

E. Medication.

1. Cardiac Tonics: Digiralis, strophanthus, caffein, strychnin.
2. Cardiac Stimulants: Camphor, alcohol, ammonia.
3. Vasodilators: Nitrites, iodids, thyroid extract.
4. Cardiac Nutritives: Iron, calcium.
5. Cardiac Emergency Drugs: Ergot, suprarenal active principle, pituitary active principle, atropin, morphin, and also some of the drugs already mentioned.

A. HYGIENE

Of all treatment for broken compensation or dilated heart, nothing equals rest in bed. Sometimes it is the only treatment that is needed. The rigidness of this rest, the length of time that it should endure, and the period at which relaxation of such rest should be allowed depend entirely on the individual patient; no rule can be established. Most of the symptoms must disappear before exercise is allowed. Perhaps a not infrequent exception to the rule is when cardiac weakness, generally a inyocarditis, develops in a patient after 50. It is not always wise to keep such a patient in bed; he may be rested and his exercise greatly restricted, but sometimes it is difficult to get him out of bed if he is kept there any length of time.

Fresh air, sunlight and anything else that makes the bedroom attractive and cheerful are essential and will aid in the recovery. The kind of nurse that is needed, trained, untrained, or a member of the family, and the amount of company or entertainment allowed must be decided for the individual patient. The patient must be distinctly individualized and the proper measures taken to give mental and physical rest, to prevent excitement, worry, melancholia and depression, and to improve the general nutrition of the body as well as the condition of the heart.

Each occurrence of broken compensation in valvular disease causes another attack of cardiac weakness to occur with less excuse than before, and several serious attacks of brokcn compensation mean before long the loss of the heart muscle's ability to recover, so that permanent dilatation occurs.

B. DIET

The food given should be just sufficient for the needs of the body; the patient should not be overfed or underfed. Any large bulk of food or liquid should not be given. Pressure on the heart causes discomfort and is therefore inadvisable. Food that causes flatulence should be avoided. Theoretically the patient should receive a little meat, an egg or two, cereal or bread, a small amount of simple vegetables, a little fruit, often milk, a sufficient amount of noneffervescent water, perhaps a cup of chocolate or cocoa, a simple dessert, sometimes ice cream; in other words, a varied, limited diet containing all the elements that are necessary to good nutrition. The diet should be varied from day to day to encourage the appetite.

It has for several years been recognized that a salt-free diet in dropsies due to disease of the kidneys is a valuable aid in causing absorption of such exudates and of preventing greater exudations. For this reason a salt-free diet is often ordered in dropsies occurring in valvular disease. Its value, however, is not so great as in kidney lesions, and if it causes hardship to the patient it should not be continued rigorously. On the other hand, large amounts of salt should of course be interdicted.

A most valuable aid in dropsies due to heart deficiencies is the so-called dry diet, which means that as little liquid as possible should be taken in order that the patient's blood may resorb the exudate in the tissues and not have the blood vessels filled or overfilled with liquid from the gastro-intestinal tract. When dropsy is present, or even when serious pendent edemas are present, the patient should drink as little liquid as possible with his meals, and between meals should sip water rather than drink a large quantity of it. This is one of tile reasons that a large milk diet, even with kidney disturbance due to cardiac lesions, is generally inadvisable. With cardiac or general circulatory weakness, a laige amount of liquid to flush out the kidneys and the whole system, so long ordered for all kidney defects or mistakes in metabolism, is a seribus mistake. The Karel diet is described in the section on cardiovascular-renal disease.

Whether it is better to give three or four small meals a day or to give a small amount of nourishment every three hours during the daytime must again depend on the individual and his ability to digest without fermentation and putrefaction or discomfort. As previously urged, not too much fluid, even milk, though it digest perfectly, should be given, as the greater the amount of fluid the greater the amount of work thrown on the heart.

C. ELIMINATION

A patient who has developed decompensation has always imperfect elimination. The skin, bowels and kidneys do not act sufficiently or well. The circulation in the skin is sluggish. The bowels are generally constipated, or there is diarrhea of the fermentative type. The amount of urine excreted is generally insufficient and likely to be concentrated and show various signs of imperfect kidney elimination. Therefore hot sponge baths, with perhaps warm alcohol rubs, are daily necessary. Gentle massage, generally in the direction to aid the circulation, will benefit the skin. If the skin is dry or in places scaly, oil rubs are of great benefit.

The bowels must be moved daily and sufficiently, but there should be no watery purging allowed or caused. If it seems advisable in the beginning of the treatment to give a calomel purge, it should be done, but such purging should ordinarily not be repeated, although occasionally a grain or two of calomel, combined with the vegetable laxatives needed, may act perfectly and without causing depression. Saline purgatives, or even laxatives, are generally not good treatment when there is cardiac weakness. The bowels should be moved by vegetable laxatives, as aloin, cascara sagrada, or some simple combination of either or both of these drugs.

Diuretics are often not satisfactory in cardiac insufficiency. The cardiac tonics which are given the patient, and the improvement of the heart from the rest in bed generally start the kidneys to secreting properly. A diuretic administered when the kidneys are suffering passive congestion from cardiac insufficiency does not generally act, and is therefore useless. If digitalis is administered, it will act as a diuretic; if caffein is deemed advisable, that will act as a diuretic. Squills may be administered, if it seems best. If for any reason the kidneys secrete less urine and become insufficient, the diet should quickly be reduced to a small amount of milk, cereal and water, and hot baths and local heat to the back should be inaugurated.

D. PHYSICAL MEASURES

Hydrotherapy is often of great value in restoring compensation by improving the surface circulation. Sponging with hot, tepid or cold water, as indicated, will increase the peripheral circulation and the normal secretions of the skin.

When compensation is perfect, in valvular lesions, more or less frequent warm baths are advisable, and often relieve the heart by equalizing the circulation. Cold sponging in the morning may be advisable, but may do harm when there is high tension; warm, not too hot, baths are of value. Anything is of value that improves the peripheral circulation and prevents the extremities from being cold.

The value of the Nauheim or other carbonated baths is perhaps often a question. They have seemed in many instances to aid in improving compensation in such patients as have been able to go abroad for the treatment. On the other hand, so many other regimens are ordered and inaugurated for these patients at these "cures" that it is hard to decide how much benefit the baths have really done. At home the artificial carbonated or carbonic acid baths do not seem to be of great value. Baths and bathing can do harm, and the decision as to which hydrotherapeutic measure shall be used can be made only after careful observation of the patient by the physician.

Gentle massage while the patient is in bed is of undoubted value; more vigorous massage is later often of value, provided there is no arteriosclerosis. As the patient grows stronger and the circulation improves, the muscles are kept in good condition during the enforced rest by massage. When properly applied, it promotes not only the venous return circulation, but also the lymphatic circulation; it often removes muscle aches and muscle tire and restlessness.

While the patient is still in bed, various resistant exercises are of value, and should be begun. These tend to prepare the patient for his later greater activities; the surprise to the heart when the patient begins to sit up and walk is not so great if he has previously taken these exercises. Later, when the patient is ambulatory, he should by gradual gradation walk a little more about the house and take a few steps of the stairs at a time, until gradually he is able to mount the whole flight. Later he should take out-door exercise, and when his heart has become compensated for ordinary work, he should be given gradually graded hill-climbing with the idea of increasing his reserve cardiac power. If it is found that these increased exertions cause him to have pain or a more rapid heart than is excusable, even after persisting for a few days, the attempt to increase this reserve power of the heart should be abandoned. There is probably, at least at that particular time, considerable myocarditis, although the heart may eventually recuperate still more. Pushing it to overexertion, however, will not accomplish improvement. Some of the simple "tests of heart strength" described under that heading may be used with these patients.

Graded exercise was first used scientifically by Oertel and Schott, and has been for years designated by their names. Modifications of their rigid rules are generally advisable.

E. MEDICATION

1. CARDIAC TONICS.-Digitalis: There is no drug that can take the place of digitalis in loss of compensation in chronic valvular disease. It acts specifically for good, and it has its greatest success in the valvular lesions that cause enlargement of the left ventricle, on which it acts the most intensely. It also acts for good on the right ventricle. It has but little action on the auricles. This is simply a question of muscle; the part that has the greatest amount of muscle will receive the greatest benefit from digitalis, and the parts that have the least, the least benefit. The heart muscle is somewhat similar to other muscles; when we attempt athletic improvement in any muscle of the body, we "train" by stimulating it moderately at first, and are careful not to overwork it; the object, then, is to train the heart muscle. For this reason large doses of digitalis should ordinarily not be given to overstimulate suddenly an overworked and

weak heart. While in some instances it has been declared that digitalis should be rapidly pushed to the full extent and then dropped for a time, careful experience shows that this method is often not tolerated, sometimes does positive harm, and has at times seemed to hasten death.

Another valuable activity of digitalis is in slowing the heart by action on the pneumogastric nerves. A dilated heart has lost more or less of its regulating mechanism; this is the cause of its irregularity and its increased rapidity. The action of digitalis in slowing the heart, giving it a longer rest, and preventing it from acting irregularly is of great value. This prolonged rest or diastole of the heart allows the circulation in the coronary arteries to become normal, and the nutrition and muscle tone of the heart improves. Digitalis also increases the blood pressure, not only by improving the activity of the heart, but also by causing some contraction of the arterioles. This feature of digitalis action in arteriosclerosis renders its use sometimes a question of careful decision. The dose of digitalis under such a condition should not be large. It may be indicated, however, and may do a great deal of good, and it does not always increase the blood pressure.

If the patient is sufficiently ill to require the best action of digitalis, an active preparation should be obtained. It was long supposed that the infusion presented activities which could not be furnished by the tincture of digitalis. This seems not to be true. The greater value of the infusion is generally because it is freshly made and active; the tincture which had been used previously in a given case was old and useless; furthermore, most physicians give a larger dose of the infusion than they ever do of the tincture. Owing to the uncertainty of the value of the digitalis leaves found in the various drug shops, however, and to variations in the preparation of the infusion, it is generally better to use a tincture of known character. The beginning dose of such a tincture should generally not be more than 5 drops, and it should not be repeated more frequently than once in eight hours. It is generally advisable, in two or three days, to increase this dose to 10 drops once in twelve hours, later perhaps to 15 drops twice a day, and still later to 20 drops once a day. This amount may then be decreased gradually, if the action is satisfactory. Enough should be given to procure results, and then the dose should be brought down to what seems sufficient and best, administered once a day. The frequence advised in the administration of this drug is because it is eliminated slowly. Its greatest action develops a number of hours after it has been taken, and then the action lasts for many hours; the administration of digitalis once in twenty-four hours is perfectly satisfactory for many patients, and more satisfactory than any more frequent administration. On the other hand, some patients do better on a smaller dose once in twelve hours. This frequence is always sufficient.

Digipuratum and digitol, a fat-free tincture, proprietary preparations accepted by the Council on Pharmacy and Chemistry for inclusion in N. N. R., may be employed. They are standardized preparations and may thus be more satisfactory than some pharmacopeial preparations of digitalis, although their claims to lessened emetic action are not borne out by recent experiments of Hatcher and Eggleston.

Digipuratum may be obtained in tubes of twelve tablets. The advice has been given for patients with loss of compensation to receive four tablets the first day, three the second, three the third, and two the fourth day. This, however, is generally an overdosage. The most that should generally be given is one of these tablets in twelve hours. Digipuratum fluid is also a valuable preparation.

Digitol is a fat-free tincture of digitalis which is physiologically standardized and which bears on each package the date of manufacture. The close is from 0.3 to 1 c.c. (5 to 15 mimims).

Digitalinum, one of the active principles of digitalis, is not very satisfactory. It may be given hypodermically, but often causes irritation, and the proper dose and its value are apt to be uncertain.

Digitoxin, another active principle of digitalis, has been declared by some investigators to be harmful, also to be liable to cause serious disturbance of a damaged heart. Other investigators have stated that it acts for good. Digitoxin does not represent the whole value of digitalis, and in broken compensation digitalis itself, or some preparation embodying the majority of its activities, should be given. Digitoxin, however, is often valuable in conditions of cardiac debility or slight weakening in patients who do not have dilated hearts or edemas. The most satisfactory dose of digalen is from 5 to 10 drops once or twice in twenty-four hours.

Digitalis should not be used when there is fatty degeneration of the heart; it should ordinarily not be used when there is arteriosclerosis, and very rarely, if ever, when it is decided that there is coronary disease. Whether digitalis should be used when there is considered to be much myocardial degeneration is a question for individualization. One can never be sure that the heart muscle is so thoroughly degenerated that no part of it would be benefited by digitalis when compensation is lost; therefore, many times, especially if other drugs have failed, small doses of digitalis should be tried, to see if the heart will respond. Large doses or frequent doses would be contraindicated.

The signs of overaction of digitalis are nausea, vomiting, a diminished amount of urine, a tight, band-like feeling around the head, perhaps occipital headache and coldness of the hands and feet, or frequently of one extremity only, combined with a feeling of numbness. The pulse is generally reduced to sixty or less a minute. Such symptoms require that digitalis be immediately stopped. They are the primary signs of cumulative action.

While many patients with ordinary dosage of digitalis may take the drug for months and years without ever showing cumulative action, other patients show this effect quickly. They are apt to be those in whom the kidneys are not perfect. The signs of such undesired action may develop slowly, as suggested by the symptoms just enumerated, or they may develop suddenly. The pulse becomes rapid and irregular, the heart action weak, there is severe backache in the region of the kidneys, a greatly diminished amount of urine, or even partial suppression, severe headache, vomiting, cold extremities and shiverings.

The treatment of such an undesired behavior of digitalis is, of course, to stop the drug immediately, give saline laxatives, hot sponging or hot baths, nitroglycerin and perhaps alcohol.

Strophanthus: Strophanthus cannot be compared with digitalis, except when the glucosid, strophanthin, is administered subcutaneously or intravenously. Strophanthus is given either in the form of the tincture, or as strophanthin. It has been shown that in neither of these forms, when the drug is administered by the stomach, is the muscle of the heart or the blood vessels much acted on. Compensation could not be restored by strophanthus. In emergencies of serious cardiac failure, strophanthin intravenously has been shown apparently to save life. It acts quickly, and its power of stimulating the heart and contracting the blood vessels lasts for many hours. It is rarely, however, that the dose should be repeated, and then not for twenty-four hours, but during that twenty-four hours the patient may be saved until other drugs which act more slowly have been absorbed, or perhaps until the emergency has passed. It probably should not be given if the patient has previously had good dosage of digitalis.

There are many, however, who believe that they obtain considerable value from the tincture of strophanthus, and there seems to be no doubt that although strophanthus, given in the form of the tincture and by the mouth, may not increase the muscle power of the heart, it many times acts as a satisfactory cardiac sedative. Under its action the patient becomes less nervous, the heart often acts more regularly, and the low blood pressure may improve. We should not be quite ready to discard the internal use of the tincture of strophanthus.

The tincture of strophanthus readily deteriorates, and the preparation ordered should be known to be a good one.

Caffein: This should not be given or allowed, even in the form of tea or coffee, to patients who have valvular lesions with perfect compensation, as it is a nervous and cardiac stimulant and may cause a heart to become irritable. It raises the blood pressure slightly, acts as a diuretic, and hence is often of great value when used medicinally. It should be ranked as a stimulotonic to the heart. It increases its activity, but gives it a little more strength. It will rarely slow a rapid heart; it will often stimulate a sluggish, slow heart; it may increase the irritability of an irritable heart. As it is a cerebral stimulant, it should not be given late in the afternoon or evening, as it may prevent sleep.

The most frequent form of caffein used is the citrated caffein. The dose is 0.1 gm. (1 1/2 grains) two or three times in the early part of the day, or 0.2 gm. (3 grains) once or twice during the morning. A few much larger doses may be given if desired. A cup of coffee may be given the patient medicinally: as a substitute for the drug, an ordinary cup of strong coffee containing between 2 and 3 grains. Other preparations of caffein may be selected if desired, or a soluble preparation may be given hypodermically.

Caffein is indicated if digitalis is contraindicated or does not act satisfactorily, and the patient is not nervously excited, but perhaps is stupid or apathetic, and also when diuresis is desired.

Strychnin: This is a valuable stimulator and heart tonic when properly used. It promotes muscular activity of the heart much as it promotes all muscular activities. It awakens nervous stimuli and nervous transmissions to normal in all sluggish nerve functions. If for these reasons the heart acts more perfectly, and the nutrition of the heart muscle improves, it acts as a cardiac tonic. Many times, by improving the action of the heart, and also by the action of the drug on the vasomotor center, the pressure in the peripheral circulation may be increased. On the other hand, strychnin in the low blood pressure of serious illness, such as pneumonia, by no means always raises the blood pressure.

It should not be forgotten that strychnin is a general nervous stimulant, especially of the spinal cord. If it makes a nervous patient more nervous, or a quiet patient restless and irritable, it is acting for harm and should be stopped, just as caffein under the same conditions should be stopped. Strychnin may cause diminished secretion of the skin. This is not frequent, but it does occur. It may prevent the patient from sleeping. If such be the fact, strychnin is not acting for good in a patient who has cardiac weakness.

INDICATIONS FOR STRYCHNIN

Strychnin is a much overused drug. It is now given for almost everything and during almost every disease. It is true that the administration of strychnin is largely due to the evolution of the age in which we are now living. We have ceased to purge and bleed and sweat, and to give large doses of aconite or veratrum viride; have ceased to starve the patient too long; we have ceased to load him with alcohol to the point of circulatory prostration, and we have recognized that he must be braced from start to finish; strychnin is the drug which has been used for this purpose, and, as stated above, overused. Strychnin given too frequently or in too large doses for a laboring heart can prevent its proper rest; the diastole is shortened and the relaxation of the heart is incomplete, its nutrition suffers, or even irregular and fibrillary contractions of a weak heart may apparently be caused. While a large dose of strychnin, even to one-twentieth grain hypodermically, may be used once in serious emergency when it is deemed the drug to use, a dose larger than one-thirtieth grain hypodermically is rarely indicated, the frequency of such a dose should seldom be more than once in six hours, and a smaller close of strychnin may act more satisfactorily.

Strychnin is indicated when the heart is acting sluggishly and the contractions seem incomplete, and when digitalis either is not indicated or is not acting perfectly. Small doses of strychnin may aid such a heart during the administration of digitalis. In many instances in which digitalis is contraindicated, strychnin is of marked value. This is typically true in fatty hearts, and may be true in arteriosclerosis, in which it often does not increase the blood pressure at all.

2. Cardiac Stimulants.—A cardiac stimulant is a drug which makes the heart beat more strongly and the frequence more nearly normal. The drugs named as cardiac stimulants, however, camphor, alcohol and ammonia, do not leave a heart better than they found it—they are not cardiac tonics.

Camphor: This is one of the best cardiac stimulants that we possess. It is a quickly acting nervous and circulatory stimulant, acting principally on the cerebrum and causing a dilation of the peripheral blood vessels. No subsequent weakness follows after a dose of camphor. Too much will make a patient wakeful, a little often quiets nervous irritability. It should be used as a cardiac stimulant during serious illness more frequently than it has been; and during the endeavor to make a noncompensating heart again compensatory camphor will often act for good. The dose is 2 teaspoonfuls of the camphor-water every three or four hours, as deemed advisable. Each teaspoonful represents a little more than one-fourth grain of camphor. The spirits of camphor, of course, may be used, if preferred.

For cardiac emergencies, ampules of sterile saturated solutions in oil are now obtainable and are valuable. Such hypodermic stimulation acts quickly, and may be repeated every half hour for several times, if the patient does not respond. The solution should be injected slowly, and as a rule intramuscularly.

Many times while other measures are being used to repair a broken compensation, camphor makes a splendid circulatory and nervous bracer. Camphor has long been used as a so-called antispasmodic in hysteric or other nervously irritable persons. It really acts as a stimulant to the highest centers of the brain, promoting more or less nervous control. Perhaps its ability to increase the peripheral circulation may be one of the reasons that it seems at times to be almost a nervous sedative by relieving internal congestion. As just stated, after the camphor action is over there is no depression. This is not true of alcohol.

Alcohol: It is of course now generally understood that alcohol is not a cardiac stimulant in the sense of its being more than momentarily helpful to a weak heart. If alcohol is pushed when a heart is in trouble, the secondary vasodilatation and more or less nerve prostration and muscle debility will cause greater circulatory weakness than before it was administered.

To obtain cardiac stimulation from alcohol it must be given in strong solutions, generally in the form of whisky or brandy, for local irritation of the mouth, esophagus and stomach; reflexly the heart is stimulated and the blood pressure rises. As soon as complete absorption has taken place, the blood pressure falls. For continuous stimulation, another dose of alcohol must be given before this depression occurs. This may be in from one to three hours. To continue such stimulation, the dose of alcohol must be increased. The future of such treatment means an alcoholic sleep with depression, alcoholic excitement which is not desired, or profound nausea and vomiting, with peripheral relaxation and cold perspiration.

Obviously none of these conditions is desirable; but in arteriosclerosis, or when the blood pressure is high and the heart labors tinder the disadvantage of contracting against an abnormal circulatory resistance, alcohol may act perfectly to relieve this kind of circulatory disturbance. In this condition the alcohol should not be given concentrated, and as soon as it is thoroughly absorbed vasodilatation occurs, peripheral circulation and therefore warmth are increased, and the heart is relieved of its extra load. In such instances, in proper doses not too frequently repeated, rarely more than 1 or 2 teaspoonfuls every three hours, alcohol is a valuable drug. Such good action of alcohol is often seen when the surface of the body is cold from chilling, or the extremities are cold from vasomotor spasm. A good-sized dose of alcohol, best given hot, equalizes the circulation and acts for good. On the contrary, it is obvious that, if the patient is cold from collapse and there is cold perspiration and very low blood pressure, alcohol is not the drug indicated, although one dose may be of benefit while other more slowly acting cardiac tonics or stimulants are being administered.

During serious prolonged illness and when the patient has not had sufficient food and is not taking sufficient food, alcohol in the form of whisky or brandy, not more than a teaspoonful every three hours, acts as a necessary food, and will more or less prevent acidosis from starvation.

It will be seen that alcohol, except possibly in a single dose occasionally, or for some special reason, is rarely indicated in decompensation.

When alcohol is administered regularly, whether during a fever process or for any other reason, if it causes a dry tongue, cerebral excitement, flushed face and a bounding pulse or if there is the odor of alcohol on the breath, the dose is too large, and alcohol is contraindicated.

Ammonia: In the form of ammonium carbonate or the aromatic spirits of ammonia, this has long been used with clinical satisfaction as a cardiac stimulant. Probably, however, it is seldom wise to use ammonium carbonate. It is exceedingly irritant, and constantly causes nausea, perhaps vomiting, and often heartburn or other gastric disturbance. It has no value over the pleasanter aromatic spirits of ammonia, which is essentially a solution of ammonium carbonate. The dose of the aromatic spirits is anywhere from a few drops to half a teaspoonful, given with plenty of water. It is thought to be a quickly acting stimulant, with an effect much like alcohol, followed by very little or no depression. It is more of a cerebral irritant than alcohol, and probably has few, if any, advantages over camphor.

When but little nutriment has been taken for some days, it may be a chemical question, since ammonium compounds so readily form and become cerebral irritants, whether any more ammonium radicals should be given the patient. This is especially true with defective kidneys. In these conditions camphor is better.

3. Vasodilators.—In various conditions of high blood pressure, arteriosclerosis and even during the sthenic stage of a fever, vasodilators may be indicated. The most important are nitrites, iodids and thyroid extracts. Alcohol, as stated above, may act as a vasodilator. Aconite and veratrum viride are now rarely indicated, although possibly aconite should be used when there is high tension and the heart is acting irritably and stormily.

If the nitrites, no preparation seems to act more satisfactorily than nitroglycerin (trinitrin, glyceryl nitratis, glonoin). Its action may not be so prolonged as other forms of nitrite, such as sodium nitrite or erythrol tetranitrate, but it is not irritant, and only a little less rapid than amyl nitrite, and although the marked dilation lasts but a short time, often apparently only for minutes, still, when frequently repeated or given a few times (from four to six) in twenty-four hours, it frequently keeps the blood pressure lower than it would be without the drug. In diseases of the heart the sudden vasodilation caused by amyl nitrite inhalations is indicated only in angina pectoris. "Then the surface of the body tends to be cold, however, when the peripheral blood pressure is increased and the heart is laboring, nitroglycerin in small doses is valuable. The dose may be from 1/400 to 1/100 grain, dissolved on the tongue or given hypodermically for quick action, or given by the mouth for more prolonged action. In sudden cardiac dyspnea nitroglycerin sometimes acts specifically, especially when there is asthma. When a drop or two of the official spirits, which is a 1 percent solution, is given on the tongue, or a soluble tablet of 1/100 grain is dissolved on the tongue, the action is almost as rapid as though the dose had been administered hypodermically. Many times when such increased peripheral circulation is desired and alcohol seems indicated, nitroglycerin in small doses will act as well. It cannot be termed a cardiac stimulant, although many times a heart acts better and the pulse is fuller and stronger after nitroglycerin than before. It should not be used, except if specially indicated, in broken compensation or in other myocardial weakness.

Iodids: These have no immediate action. The vasorelaxation that often occurs from iodid is quite likely due to the stimulation of the thyroid gland by the iodin, and the thyroid gland secretes a vasodilating substance. Small doses of iodid, however, when indicated in various kinds of sclerosis, have seemed to lower blood pressure. While large doses may have more of this actioli, they are not now under consideration, and large doses are rarely indicated. Too mach iodid has been given for many conditions. If the indications for an iodid are present, such as sclerosis anywhere, or unabsorbed inflammatory products, exudation in or around the heart, or an apparent insufficiency of the thyroid, from 0.1 to 0.2 gm. (1 1/2 to 3 grains) once or twice in twenty-four hours, after meals, is all that is required to give the action desired, and the circulation is benefited. It is sometimes a question whether small doses of iodid are not actually stimulant to the heart, possibly through the action on the thyroid gland.

Thyroid Extract: In slow hearts and in sluggish circulation, often in old age, quite frequently in arteriosclerosis and in every condition of insufficient thyroid secretion (these instances are frequent), small doses of thyroid extract will benefit the circulation. Its satisfactory action is to increase the cardiac activity, slightly lower the blood pressure, and increase the peripheral circulation and the health of the skin. If it causes tachycardia, nervous excitement, sleeplessness or loss of weight, it is doing harm and the dose is too large, or it is not indicated. The dose for the cardiac action desired is a tablet representing from 1/2 to 1 grain of the active substalice of the thyroid gland, given once a day, continued for a long period.

When an improved peripheral circulation is desired, and especially when a reduction of the pressure in the heart is desired and a diminished amount of blood in overfilled arteries is indicated, the value of the sitzbath, hot foot-baths, warm liquids (not hot) in the stomach, and warm, moist applications to the abdomen should all be remembered.

4. Cardiac Nutritives.—Iron: Nothing is of more value to a weakened heart muscle, when the nutrition is low, the patient anemic, and the iron of the food not properly metabolized, than tonic doses of some iron salt. It has frequently been repeated, but should constantly be reiterated, that there is no physiologic reason or therapeutic excuse for the patient to pay a large amount of money for some organic iron preparation.

Small doses of an inorganic salt act perfectly, and nothing will act better. As previously suggested, a drop or two of the tincture of iron, a grain or two of the reduced iron, or 2 or 3 grains of saccharated ferric oxid, given once or twice in twenty-four hours, is all the iron the body needs from the points of view of the blood and the heart.

Calcium: It has lately been learned that calcium is an element which a heart needs for perfect activity. Many patients who are ill lose their calcium, and they may not receive a sufficient amount of it unless milk is given them. Even if such patients are taking milk, the heart and the whole general condition sometimes such; to improve when calcium is added to the diet. It may be given either in the form of lime water, calcium lactate or calcium glycerophosphate. If a medium-sized dose is given three or four times in twenty-four hours, it is sufficient and will often act for good.

Whether calcium can do harm in a chronic endocarditis or an arteriosclerosis to offset the value that it seems to have in quieting the nervous system and in being of value to a weak or nervously irritable heart is a question which has not been decided. Theoretically lime should not be given when there is a tendency to calcification, or when a patient is past middle age. Lime seems to be essential to youth, and to the welfare of nervous patients.

EMERGENCIES

5. Cardiac Emergency Drugs.—Besides some of the drugs already mentioned (such as camphor hypodermically, nitroglycerin when indicated, strophanthin hypodermically or intravenously, caffein

and strychnin), often ergot, suprarenal vasopressor principle, pituitary vasopressor principle, atropin and morphin should be considered.

When there is low blood pressure, venous stasis, pulmonary congestion, cyanosis and a laboring, failing heart, intramuscular injections of ergot, with or without coincident venesection, may be the most valuable method of combating the condition. Life has been saved in this kind of sudden acute cardiac failure in valvular disease. When venesection is not indicated in certain conditions of low blood pressure and heart failure, ergot has saved life. It causes contraction of the blood vessels and seems to tone the heart. Incidentally it quiets the central nervous system. If the blood pressure is much increased by it, the ergot should not be repeated, as too much work should not be thrown on the heart muscle. Often, however, it may be administered intramuscularly with advantage in aseptic preparation as offered in ampules, at the rate of one ampule every three hours for two or three times, and then once in six hours for a few times, the future frequency depending on the indications.

Epinephrin and Pituitary Extract: The blood pressure-raising substance of the suprarenals or of the pituitary gland (hypophysis cerebri) has been much used in heart failure. These substances certainly would not be indicated in high blood pressure; they are indicated in low blood pressure. They have been given intravenously; they are frequently given hypodermically. They often act rapidly when a solution in proper dose is dropped on the tongue. The blood pressure rise from epinephrin is quickly over; that from the pituitary extract lasts longer. In large doses, or when it is too frequently repeated, epinephrin depresses the respiration. Pituitary extract acts as a diuretic. Sterilized solutions of both, put up in ampules ready for hypodermic medication, are obtainable, the strength offered generally being 1 part of the active principle to 10,000 of the solution. Hypodermic tablets of epinephrin may also be obtained. Stronger solutions of 1 part to 1,000 may be dropped on the tongue, or tablets may be dissolved on the tongue. The blood pressure is temporarily raised and the heart stimulated by these treatments, but epinephrin is not used so often for cardiac failure as it was a short time ago.

The most satisfactory action, especially from the epinephrin, is from small doses frequently repeated. Sometimes in serious emergencies it has been found to be of value when given intravenously in physiologic saline solution. The close, of course, should be very small. In circulatory weakness in acute illness, epinephrin has been given regularly, a few drops (perhaps the most frequent dose is 5) of a 1: 1,000 solution, on the tongue, once in six hours. Such a dosage may be of value, and certainly is better than the administration of too much strychnin. Much larger or more frequent doses are likely, as just stated, to depress the respiration.

Besides the small amount of blood pressure-raising substance secreted by the hypophysis cerebri. it has not been shown that any other gland of the body furnishes vasopressor substance except the suprarenals.

Atropin: When there is great cardiac weakness, atropin may be used to advantage. The dose is from 1/200 to 1/150 grain hypodermically, not repeated in many hours. It will whip up a flagging heart, more or less increase the blood pressure, cause cerebral awakening, and may often be of value. If there is any idiosyncrasy against atropin, if the throat and mouth are made intensely dry, or if there is serious flushing or cerebral excitement, the dose should not be repeated.

Morphin: This would rarely be considered as an emergency drug in cardiac weakness. A small dose of it, not more than one-eighth grain, especially if combined with atropin, will often quiet and brace a weak heart, especially when there is cardiac pain. Just which drug or drugs should be used and just which are not indicated can never be specifically outlined in a textbook, a lecture or a paper. The decision can be made only at the bedside, and then mistakes, many times unavoidable, are often made.

In all conditions of shock with cardiac failure, the blood vessels of the abdomen and splauclinic system are dilated, and more or less of the blood of the body is lost in these large veins, and the peripheral and cerebral blood pressure fails. The advantage in such a condition of firm abdominal bandages, and of raising the foot of the bed or of raising the feet and legs, need only be mentioned to be understood.

It is a pretty good working rule, in cardiac failure, not to do too much. On the other hand, life is frequently saved by proper treatment, and the physician repeatedly saves life as surely as does the surgeon with his knife.

CONVALESCENCE

When compensation has been restored, the patient may be allowed gradually to resume his usual habits and work, provided these habits are sensible, and the work is not one requiring severe muscular exertion. Careful rules and regulations must be laid down for him, depending on his age and the condition of his arteries, kidneys and heart muscle. It should be remembered that a patient over 40, who has had broken compensation, is always in more dancer of a recurrence of this weakness than one who is younger, as after 40 the blood pressure normally increases in all persons, and this normal increase may be just too much for a compensating heart which is overcoming all of the handicap that it can withstand. Such patients, then, should be more carefully restricted in their habits of life, and also should have longer and more frequent periods of rest.

The avoidance of all sudden exertion in any instance in which compensation has just been restored is too important not to be frequently repeated. The child must be prevented from hard playing, even running with other children, to say nothing of bicycle riding, tennis playing, baseball, football, rowing, etc. The older boy and girl may need to be restricted in their athletic pleasures, and dancing should often be prohibited. Young adults may generally, little by little, assume most of their ordinary habits of life; but carrying heavy weights upstairs, going up more than one flight of stairs rapidly, hastening or running on the street for any purpose, and exertion, especially after eating a large meal, must all be prohibited. Graded physical exercise or athletic work, however, is essential for the patients' future health, and first walking and later more energetic exercise may be advisable.

These patients must not become chilled, as they are liable to catch cold, and a cold with them must not be neglected, as coughing or lung congestions are always more serious in valvular disease. Their feet and hands, which are often cold, should be properly clothed to keep them warm. Chilling of the extremities drives the blood to the interior of the body, increases congestion there, and by peripheral contraction raises the general blood pressure. A weak heart generally needs the blood pressure strengthened, but a compensating heart rarely needs an increase in peripheral blood pressure, and any great increase from any reason is a disadvantage to such a heart. The patient should sleep in a well ventilated room, but should not suffer the severe exposures that are advocated for pulmonary tuberculosis, as severe chilling of the body must absolutely be avoided.

The peripheral circulation is improved, the skin is kept healthy, the general circulation is equalized, and the heart is relieved by a proper frequency of warm baths. Cold baths are generally inadvisable, whether the plunge, shower or sponging; very hot baths are inadvisable on account of causing a great deal of faintness; while warm baths are not stimulating and are sedative. The Turkish and Russian bath should be prohibited. They are never advisable in cardiac disease. With kidney insufficiency, body hot-air treatment (body-baking), carefully supervised, may greatly benefit a patient who has no dilatation of the heart and who has no serious broken compensation. Surfbathing, and, generally, sea-bathing and lake-bathing are not advisable. The artificial sea-salt baths and carbon dioxid baths may do some good, but they do not lower the general blood pressure so surely as has been advocated, and probably no great advantage is apt to be derived from such baths. If a patient cannot properly exercise, massage should be given him intermittently.

Any systemic need should be supplied. If the patient is anemic, he should receive iron. If he has no appetite, he should be encouraged by bitter tonics. If sleep does not come naturally, it must be induced by such means as do not injure the heart.

Perhaps there is no better place in this series on diseases of the heart to discuss the diet in general and the resort treatment than at this point, as the question is one of moment after convalescence from a broken compensation, at which time every means must be inaugurated to establish a reserve heart strength to overcome the daily emergencies of life.

DIET AND BATHS IN HEART DISEASE

The diet in cardiac diseases has already incidentally been referred to. The decision as to what a patient ought to eat or drink must often be modified by just what the patient will do, and, as we all know, it is absolutely necessary to make some concessions in order for him to aid us in hastening his own recovery or in preventing him from having relapses. Consequently, we cannot be dogmatic with most patients with chronic heart disease. Parents should be prohibited from allowing children or adolescents with heart disease to drink tea, coffee or any alcoholic stimulant. The young boy and young man must absolutely be prohibited from indulging in tobacco at all. There is no excuse for allowing these stimulants or foods in such cases. If the patient is older and has been accustomed to tea and coffee, one cup of coffee in the morning may be allowed, provided a decaffeinated coffee is not found satisfactory. Whether a small cup of coffee or a cup of tea is allowed at noon is again a matter for individualization; they should rarely be allowed after the noon meal. In a patient who has been accustomed to alcohol regularly (generally an older patient), careful judgment should be used in deciding whether or not a small amount of alcohol daily should be allowed. It should never be in large amounts, even of a dilute alcohol like beer; it may be a weak wine; it may be a small amount of diluted whisky, if seems best. Ordinarily the patient is better without it. If he is used to smoking and a small amount does not raise the blood pressure much, it may do him no harm to smoke a small mild cigar once or twice a clay. On the other hand, if a hard smoker suddenly has heart failure, whether from exertion, from chronic disease or from acute illness, a small amount of smoking is of advantage as it tends to remove cardiac irritability, to raise the blood pressure, and actually to quiet and improve the circulation. It is unwise during acute circulatory failure to take tobacco away entirely from a chronic tobacco user.

The character of the food which each patient should receive depends on his blood pressure and his age. The older person with a tendency to high blood pressure should have the protein (especially meat) reduced in amount, as any putrefaction in the intestine with absorption of products of such maldigestion irritates the blood vessels, raises the blood pressure, and injuries the kidneys. On the other hand, a young patient should receive a sufficient meat diet rather than be overloaded with vegetables and starches, to the easy production of fermentation and gas. Flatulence from any cause must be avoided. It dilates the stomach and intestines, causing them to press on the diaphragm, so that the heart and respiration are interfered with. Also, an increased abdominal pressure, especially if there is any edema or dropsy, is bad for the circulation. A distended, tense abdomen is serious in cardiac failure. On the other hand, a flaccid, flabby, lax abdomen should be well bandaged in cardiac failure with low blood pressure.

Children do well on a milk diet, but it should be remembered that excessive amounts of any liquid, even milk and water, are inadvisable, if the circulation is poor and there is a tendency to dropsy. It has been recommended at times to limit a patient's diet for a week or so to a small amount of milk, not more than a quart in twenty-four hours. If such a patient is in bed and does not require carbohydrates, sugars or stronger proteins or more fat, such a restricted diet may aid in establishing circulatory equilibrium, although he will lose in nutrition. The excretory organs are relieved by the decreased amount of excretory product, the digestive system is rested and the circulation is improved. Such a limited diet should not be tried longer than a week, but it may be the turning point of circulatory improvement.

The ordinary diet for a convalescing heart patient should be small in bulk, of good nutritive value, and should represent all the different elements for nutrition. This means a small amount of meat, once a day to older patients, twice a day to those who work hard or for young patients; such vegetables as do not cause indigestion with the particular patient, and these must be individualized; such fruits as are readily digested, especially cooked fruits; generally plenty of butter, cream, olive oil if the nutrition is low, and milk, depending on the age of the patient or the ease with which it is digested. Soups, on account of their bulk and low nutritive value, should be avoided. Anything that causes indigestion, such as fried foods, hot bread, oatmeal or any other gummy, sticky, gelatinous cereal should be avoided; also spices, sauces and strong condiments. Anything that is recognized as especially loaded with nuclein and xanthin bodies, such as liver, sweetbreads and kidneys, should be prohibited, as tending to cause uric acid disturbance; and the more tendency to gout or uric acid malmetabolism the more irritated are the arteries and the more disturbed the blood pressure. Sugars should be used moderately unless the patient is thin and feels cold, in which case more may be given, provided there are no signs of gout or disturbed sugar metabolism. Sugar is at times a good stimulant food. Very cold and very hot drinks or food should be avoided.

Many times these patients have a diminished hydrochloric acid secretion, and such patients thrive on 5 drops of dilute hydrochloric acid in water, three times a day, after meals. When their nutrition has improved and the digestion becomes perfect, hydrochloric acid will generally be sufficiently secreted and the medication may be stopped.

If the patient is overweight, this obesity must be reduced, as nothing more interferes with the welfare of the heart than overweight and overfat. In these cases the diet should be that required for the condition. If there are edemas, or a tendency to edemas, the decision should be made whether salt (sodium chlorid) should be removed from the diet. Unless there is kidney defect, probably it need not be omitted, and a long salt-free diet is certainly not advisable. This salt-free diet has been recommended not only in nephritis and heart disease, but also in diabetes insipidus and in epilepsy. It is of value if there is edema in nephritis; it is of doubtful value in heart disease; it is rarely of value in diabetes insipidus; and in epilepsy its value consists probably in allowing the bromid that may be administered to have better activity in smaller doses, the bromin salt being substituted in the metabolism for the chlorin salt.

THE RESORT TREATMENT OF CHRONIC HEART DISEASE

In line with the continued growing popularity of special resorts and special cures for different types of disease, resort or sanatorium treatment for chronic heart disease has grown to considerable popularity during the last twenty years or more. The most popular of these resorts owe their success to the personality of the physicians, who have made heart disease a life study.

Perhaps the most noted of these resorts for the cure of heart disease is that at Bad Nauheim, Germany, which was inaugurated by Dr. August Schott and Prof. Theodore Schott, and is now conducted by the latter, Dr. August Schott having died about fifteen years ago. Hundreds of patients and many physicians have testified to the value and benefit of the treatment carried out at this institution.

The method of treatment largely employed at these heart resorts is to withdraw all, or nearly all, of the active drugs that the patient may be taking, and to substitute physical and physiologic methods of therapy. These include bathing, regulation of the diet, and exercise. This exercise consists of two varieties: exercise of the muscles against the resistance of an attendant, and exercise by walking on inclined planes or up hills. The treatment is aimed at chronic heart disease, to develop a greater cardiac reserve strength; the whole object of the treatment is to strengthen the myocardium, either in conditions of its debility or in conditions of diminished compensation in valvular disease. Any treatment that will develop a reserve heart strength to be called on in emergencies, more or less similar to the reserve strength of a normal heart, tends to prolong the patient's life and health.

Patients with acute heart failure or acute loss of compensation, with more or less serious edemas, should rarely take the risk of traveling any distance to be treated at an institution. As a general rule they are better treated for a few weeks or months at home. After the broken compensation is repaired, a reserve strength of the heart may well be developed by a visit to one of these institutions, if the patient can afford it.

The Oertel treatment consists chiefly in diminishing the fluids taken into the body, and in graduated mountain climbing. By diminishing the fluids taken, the work of the heart is diminished, as the blood vessels are not overfilled and may be even underfilled. The diet is carefully regulated with the object of removing all superfluous fat from the body. The third leg of the tripod of the Oertel treatment is the gradually increasing hill and mountain climbing to educate the heart by graded muscular training to become strong, perfectly compensatory, and later to develop a reserve strength. This particular cure is especially adapted to the obese, who have weakened heart muscles.

NAUHEIM BATHS

At Nauheim, under the direction of Dr. Theodore Schott, baths form an important part of the treatment. These baths are of two kinds, the saline and the carbonic acid. The medicinal constituents of the saline bath are sodium chlorid and calcium chlorid, the strength of each varying from 2 to 3 percent The baths at first arc given at a temperature of 95 F., and as the patient becomes used to them and can take them without discomfort, the temperature is gradually reduced. The patient remains in the bath from five to ten minutes. After the bath he is dried with towels and rubbed until the cutaneous circulation becomes active. He must then lie down for an hour. These baths are repeated for two or three days, and are omitted on the third and fourth days, to be resumed on the following day. After a few baths have been taken, the carbon dioxid baths are commenced, beginning with a small quantity of the gas which is later gradually increased. This course of baths should be continued from four to eight weeks. Unless there is some special reason for taking them at some other period of the year, they are taken more advantageously during the warm months.

Besides the baths, all important part of the treatment at Nauheim consists in the exercises against resistance. These are usually given an hour or more aftcr a bath, and are taken with great deliberation; their effect is carefully watched by an intelligent attendant so that no harm may be done by the exercise.

During this treatment the food is, of course, carefully regulated with the aim of giving a mixed, sufficient, easily digestible and easily assimilated diet. All highly seasoned dishes, all effervescent drinks and anything that tends to cause gas in the stomach and intestines are prohibited. Coffee and tea are not allowed, except coffee without caffein; and it may be noted that it has recently been shown that caffein is one of the surest of drugs to raise the blood pressure, and is therefore generally not desirable when the heart muscle requires strengthening. Because of its tendency to raise blood pressure and weaken cardiac muscle, tobacco is entirely forbidden at Nauheim, except in a few individual instances, and then the amount allowed is a minimum one. Large amounts of liquid are not allowed because they distend the stomach, raise the blood pressure and increase the pumping work of the heart.

One of the greatest advantages of the treatment at an institution like Nauheim is the general hopeful spirit instilled into the patients, who are so many times seriously depressed by the knowledge of a heart weakness and the realization of their physical inability to do what other persons are able to do. Also, it is of great value to send a patient to a resort where the climate is good and the scenery is lovely and soothing. No disease, perhaps, needs cheerfulness and pleasantness and lack of anxiety, or frets more than does cardiac weakness. A tuberculous patient may sit on a mountain top with snow blowing about him, and recover; a heart patient must have sunshine and comfort.

The results of such sanatorium treatment of heart disease are often evident not only to the patient by an increase of general muscle strength, the ability to do ordinary things and perhaps even sustain muscular effort without dyspnea and cardiac discomfort, but also to the physician by the physical signs. The contraction of the heart becomes stronger and the normal sounds more decided; murmurs which were entirely due to dilated ventricles and insufficiency disappear, while the permanent murmurs may become louder from a more forceful, normal action of the heart muscle. The pulse becomes slower, and the blood pressure, from being too low, becomes normal for the age of the individual. The heart will often also actually decrease in size, and the apex beat become localized rather than diffuse, The liver becomes reduced in size; the urine is less concentrated, and if there were traces of albumin after exertion, these disappear.

It should perhaps be emphasized that not a little benefit from these resort treatments may be due to the withdrawal of unnecessary drugs. Many heart patients are overdrugged.

This sort of treatment is contraindicated in some kinds of heart disease, as heart weakness due to arteriosclerosis with high blood pressure, to aneurysm of the thoracic or abdominal aorta, and to nephritis.

So many heart patients have been improved by the Nauheim treatment that the question arises as to whether the treatment can be conducted at home or in a sanatorium near home, when the patient is unable to go to this resort; that is to say, Can we establish this treatment for the majority of patients who have chronic heart disease? Of course, even at home, the sodium chlorid and calcium chlorid baths may be given, and one may obtain the salts all prepared to make the carbon dioxid bath; the exercises may be given, and walking on various ascending grades may be inaugurated. All patients will be more or less benefited, provided they will carry out the treatment. Unfortunately, the surroundings at a patient's home are generally adverse to perpetuating these treatments long enough to develop the muscular strength of the heart to the reserve desired. If a patient appears pretty well, especially if he is stimulated by his family to believe that he is well, he thinks the continuation of the treatment entirely unnecessary, and unless he goes to a resort where he sees other patients with similar conditions able to do what he is not able to do, and therefore is stimulated to acquire their ability by the treatment outlined, he will not follow his physician's directions. There are several sanatoriums in this country where the diet, hydrotherapy and exercise necessary for developing heart strength are carried out, and patients are sent to some of them with great advantage.

It has been found that these stimulant baths do not act well in mitral stenosis, if the left ventricle is small. If the left ventricle is unable to receive and therefore send out into the systemic circulation sufficient blood to dilate the peripheral capillaries under the irritation of the baths or the vasodilator effects of the baths, the bath treatment does harm instead of good. A patient who has mitral stenosis and also a small left ventricle will be found to be poorly developed, badly nourished, and to have poor peripheral circulation.

As elsewhere stated, the improvised carbon dioxid bath, to stimulate the skin so as to reduce the blood pressure, is not satisfactory. Other methods of reducing blood pressure, when it is too high, are much more effective.

HEART DISEASE IN CHILDREN AND DURING PREGNANCY

A common characteristic in a large proportion of middle-aged or old patients with heart disease is the presence of degenerative changes in the myocardium, the valves, or the arteries of the heart. In children, on the other hand, the most common disturbances of the heart are acute inflammations affecting its different structures, and due in most instances to acute infections. Myocarditis and endocarditis occur frequently, and pericarditis occasionally. As in adults, rheumatism is the most common cause of inflammation of the structures of the heart, but rheumatism causes inflammation of the heart much more frequently in children than in adults. Besides this infection, the most frequent causes of inflammation of the heart in children are diphtheria, scarlet fever, typhoid fever, measles and influenza, with the frequency, perhaps, in the order named. Diphtheria frequently gives rise to myocarditis, which results in dilatation of the heart. This may occur in the second or third week of the course of the disease, and even up to the eighth and tenth week from the beginning of the disease. The myocarditis due to diphtheria is not always the cause of sudden death occurring during the disease, as such a fatal result may be due to paralysis of nervous origin. In scarlet fever, inflammation of the heart may be due directly to the poison of the disease, or it may be secondary to a nephritis which is so frequent a complication of scarlet fever. It is probable that the inflammation of the skin in scarlet fever, preventing normal secretion, may be a cause of a sometimes increased blood pressure and also of the nephritis, both of which conditions may predispose to the cardiac complication. Erysipelas may cause acute inflammation of the heart, perhaps for the same reason.

A certain proportion of cardiac diseases in children, especially endocarditis, seems to be due to a general septic infection which results in the so-called septic, infectious or malignant endocarditis. There is sometimes a tendency in certain children, and perhaps in certain families, for the heart to become readily infected during an infectious disease, more than in other children who suffer from the same disease. Sometimes the heart becomes inflamed in rheumatic children without any joint affection occurring; the inflammation in the heart may be the only manifestation of the disease.

This etiology of cardiac affections of children indicates the directions in which therapeutic efforts should be aimed. In children who are under the more or less constant care of the family physician, the possibility of the occurrence of some cardiac affection should be borne in mind, especially in children in families which are known to be affected with what may be called a rheumatic diathesis—families in which several members have suffered from rheumatism. It is reasonable to suppose that children who are delicate and feeble, who do not have sufficient fresh air, who do not take sufficient exercise, and who are not properly fed are more liable to be affected with cardiac complications in the presence of infectious diseases than children who have had plenty of fresh air, an abundance of exercise and a sufficient amount of proper food.

At the present day it is hardly necessary to insist on the importance of giving every child an adequate amount of fresh air. It is possible, however, that this gospel has been overworked, and it is not infrequently necessary to caution some parents that there is danger of impairing their children's health by too much exposure. The old ideas of the influence of exposure to cold and dampness in the production of rheumatism have not yet been so far abandoned that we can entirely neglect the possibility of rheumatism being developed, at least, by the exposure to cold winds and dampness of children who are otherwise predisposed to this disease. It is possible that the enormously increasing number of children with adenoids and enlarged tonsils, who need operative measures for their removal, may have these conditions aggravated by too much exposure to the inclemency of variable, harsh weather.

It is not necessary to state that proper exercise develops the heart, as it does all the other muscles; but at the same time it is necessary to caution parents against allowing their children to indulge in too violent and too prolonged exercise. Young children probably stop often enough in their play not to overwork their hearts. Older boys and girls, especially boys, are inclined to take too severe athletics, such as long-distance running, competitive rowing, violent football and rapid cycling. It should be emphasized to school-masters, gymnasium teachers and athletic trainers that a boy who is larger than he should be at his age has not the circulatory ability that the older boy of the same size has. The overgrown boy has all he can do to carry his bulk around at the speed of his age and youth. The addition of competitive labor overreaches his reserve heart power, and he readily acquires a strained, injured heart. On the other hand, moderate indulgence in walking, baseball, swimming, rowing and golf should be commended. It is not exactly the exercise that does him the harm, it is the competitive element in it. Until a boy is well developed in his internal reserve strength, he should not compete with other boys who are better developed. His pride makes him do himself injury.

Dietetic fads are so prevalent today that there is danger that many children will not receive an adequate amount of nutriment, that they will be fed an excess of such foods as are likely to produce damage to their constitutions, or that they will be given food which does not contain all the different elements of nutrition to satisfy their economy and their growth. While it is now generally acknowledged that an excess of meat is not beneficial to any one, on the other hand a moderate amount is necessary for individuals who are working or are mentally active, especially for growing children. Also a too great limitation of the child's diet to farinaceous foods, and especially the allowance of too much sugar and sugar-producing food, is liable to encourage the development of rheumatism. A mixed diet, not excessive in amount, and prepared so that it will be digested without difficulty, is most useful, and it should include in suitable proportions meat, milk, eggs, vegetables, starches and fruit. These should all be taken at regular intervals, thoroughly chewed, and should not be taken in excess.

If a child has had an attack of heart inflammation, a myocarditis or an endocarditis, greater care should be taken of him not only when he is well but especially when he becomes ill of any other disease. If the child has had a rheumatic inflammation of the heart, or has had rheumatism without such a complication, it is considered by some clinicians wise to give a week's treatment with salicylates at intervals of three or four months, for two or three years, perhaps. It is hard to determine how much value this prophylactic treatment has. If the child's surroundings cannot be changed and lie is subjected to the same conditions of possible reinfection, it may be a wise precaution, much like the prophylactic administration of quinin in malarial regions. If a child has developed a cardiac inflammation during any disease, the treatment is that previously outlined.

An important part of prophylaxis and treatment of a cardiac affection during the course of any disease is the prevention of serious anemia. During sickness the patient is liable to become more or less anemic, but the administration of iron, in the manner previously suggested, during the course of the disease, and especially during rheumatism, will prevent the anemia becoming rapid or severe.

CARDIAC DISEASE IN PREGNANCY

It is so serious a thing for a woman with valvular lesion or other cardiac defect to become pregnant that no young woman with heart disease should be allowed to marry. Perhaps every normal heart during pregnancy hypertrophies somewhat to do the extra work thrown on it, but it may easily become weakened and show serious disturbance as its work grows harder and the distention of the abdomen and the upward pressure on the diaphragm increase. This pressure perhaps generally displaces the apex of the heart to the left and causes the heart to lie a little more horizontal. If the patient is normal, there may be a gradually increasing blood pressure all through the months of pregnancy, and if the kidneys are at all disturbed this pressure is increased, and there is, of course, much increased resistance to the circulation during labor. The better the heart acts, the less likely are edemas of the legs during pregnancy. It is thus readily seen that pregnancy is a serious thing for a damaged heart. The reserve strength of the heart muscle, as has been previously stated, is much less in valvular compensation than that of the normal heart, and this reserve force is easily overcome by the pregnancy, and loss of compensation occurs with all of its usual symptoms.

The most serious lesion a woman may have, as far as pregnancy is concerned, is mitral stenosis. An increased abdnominal pressure interferes with her lung capacity, and her lungs are already over-congested. The left ventricle may be small with mitral stenosis, and therefore her general systemic circulation poor. For those two reasons mitral stenosis should absolutely prohibit pregnancy. While many women with well compensated valvular disease go through pregnancy without serious trouble, still, as stated above, they should be advised never to marry. If they do marry, or if the lesion develops after marriage, warning should be given of the seriousness of pregnancies.

If a woman becomes pregnant while there are symptoms or signs of broken compensation, there can be no question, medically or morally, of the advisability of evacuating the uterus. The same ruling is true if during pregnancy the heart fails, compensation is broken, and the usual symptoms of such heart weakness develop, provided a period of rest in bed, with proper treatment, has shown that the heart will not again compensate. Under such a condition delay should not be too long, as the heart may become permanently disabled. If, during pregnancy in a patient with a damaged heart, albuminuria develops and the blood pressure is increased, showing kidney insufficiency, there can be no question of delay, from every point of view, and labor must be precipitated; the uterus must be emptied to save the mother's life.

If a pregnant woman is known to have a degenerative condition of the myocardium, or arteriosclerosis, the danger from the pregnancy is serious, and the pregnancy should rarely be allowed to continue.

Even if no serious symptoms occur during the term of the pregnancy, and the heart continues to compensate sufficiently for its defect, labor should never be allowed to be prolonged. The tension thrown on the heart during labor is always severe, and has not infrequently caused acute heart failure by causing acute dilatation, and in these damaged hearts tediousness and severe, intense exertion should not be allowed. Proper anesthetics and proper instrumentation should be inaugurated early.

Patients who have successfully passed through the danger of pregnancy with cardiac lesions, possibly relieved by radical treatments, should be warned against ever again becoming pregnant. If this warning does not prevent future pregnancies, the family physician and his consultant must decide just what it is proper to do. It is to be understood that no uterus should ever be emptied until one or more consultants have approved of such treatment.

Sometimes serious heart weakness develops during the later weeks of pregnancy, requiring the patient to remain in bed and receive every advantage which rest, proper care and well judged medicinal treatment will give the circulation.

If the heart is weak and there have been signs of myocardial weakness or loss of compensation, the sudden loss of abdominal pressure after delivery may allow the blood vessels of the abdomen to become so overfilled as to cause serious cerebral anemia and cardiac paralysis. Therefore in such cases a tight bandage must immediately be applied, and it has even been suggested that a weight, as a bag of sand weighing several pounds, be placed temporarily on the abdomen. The greatest possible care should be given these women during and after labor.

Acute dilatation is not an infrequent cause of death during ordinary labor, and is more apt to occur in these cardiac patients. If signs of acute dilatation of the heart occur, with associated pulmonary edema, venesection (especially if there has not been much uterine hemorrhage), with the coincident intramuscular injection of one or two syringefuls of aseptic ergot, will often be found to be life- saving treatment. Septic infections after parturition are prone to cause endocarditis and myocarditis, and a malignant endocarditis may develop from uterine infection or uterine putridity.

DEGENERATIONS

CORONARY SCLEROSIS

While disease of the coronary arteries may occur without general arteriosclerosis, it is so frequently associated with it that it is necessary to give a brief description of the general disease. Arteriosclerosis or arteriocapillary fibrosis is really a physiologic process naturally accompanying old age, of which it is a part or the cause, and it should be considered a pathologic condition only when it occurs prematurely. It may, however, occur at almost any age after 30, and is beginning to be frequent between 40 and 50. In rare instances it may occur between 20 and 30, and even in childhood and youth. It is much more frequent in men than in women. Its most common cause is hypertension; in fact, hypertension generally precedes it. The most frequent cause of hypertension today is the strenuousness of life, the next most frequent cause being the toxins circulating in the blood from overeating, overdrinking, overuse of tobacco and the overuse of caffein in the form of coffee, tea or caffein drinks. Another common cause of arteriosclerosis occurring too early is the occurrence of some serious infection in a person, typhoid fever and sepsis being most frequent. Syphilis is a frequent cause, especially of that form of arteriosclerosis which shows the greatest amount of disease in the aorta. Mercury used in the treatment of syphilis is more liable, however, than syphilis to be the cause of arteriosclerosis. Although this drug, even with the arsenic injections now in vogue, is necessary for the cure of syphilis, it probably tends to raise the blood pressure by irritating the kidneys and by diminishing the thyroid secretion, both of these occurrences predisposing to arteriosclerosis. From the fact that lead poisoning causes an increased blood pressure, lead is a probable cause of arteriosclerosis. With the greater knowledge of the danger of poisoning possessed by those who work in lead, chronic lead poisoning is becoming rare, as evidenced by the lessening frequency of wrist drop and lead colic.

Chronic nephritis is often a coincident disease, but the causes of the arteriosclerosis and the nephritis are generally the same. Alcohol, except as a part of overeating and as a disturber of the digestion, is perhaps not a direct cause of arteriosclerosis, as alcohol is a vasodilator. Hard physical labor and severe athletic work may cause arteriosclerosis to develop, and it is liable to develop in the arteries of the parts most used.

Hypertension is generally a prelude to arteriosclerosis, and everything which tends to increase tension promotes the disease; everything which tends to diminish tension more or less inhibits the disease. Therefore a subsecretion of the thyroid predisposes to arteriosclerosis, and increased secretion of the suprarenals predisposes to arteriosclerosis, the thyroid furnishing vasodilator substance and the suprarenals vasopressor substance to the blood. Furthermore. if these secretions are abnormal, protein metabolism is more or less disturbed.

While arteriosclerosis often occurs coincidently with gout, and gout apparently may be a cause of arteriosclerosis, still the two diseases are widely dissociated, and the causes are not the same.

Although the arterial pressure has been high before arteriosclerosis developed, and may remain high for some time in the arteries, unless the heart fails, the distal peripheral pressure, as in the fingers and toes, may be poor in spite of the high blood pressure. When the left heart begins to fail, pendent edema readily occurs.

PATHOLOGY

The pathology of arteriosclerosis is a thickening and diminishing elasticity of the arteries, beginning with the inner coat and gradually spreading and involving all the coats, the larger arteries often developing calcareous deposits or thickened cartilaginous plates—an atheroma. If the thickening of the walls of the smaller vessels advances, their caliber is diminished, and there may even be complete obstruction (endarteritis obliterans). On the other hand, some arteries, especially if the calcareous deposits are considerable, may become weakened in spots and dilation may occur, causing either smaller or larger aneurysms.

Histologically the disease is a connective tissue formation beginning first as a round-cell infiltration in the subendothelial layer of the intima. This process does not advance homogeneously; one side of an artery may be more affected than the other, and the lumen may be narrowed at one side and not at the other, allowing the artery to expand irregularly from the force of the heart beat. As the disease continues, the internal elastic layer is lost, the muscular coat begins to atrophy, and then small calcareous granules may begin to be deposited, which may form into plates. In the large arteries, the advance of the process differs somewhat. There may be more actual inflammatory signs, fatty degeneration may occur, and even a necrosis may take place.

However generally distributed arteriosclerosis is, in some regions the disease is more advanced than in others, and in those regions the most serious symptoms will occur. The regions which can stand the disease least well are the brain and coronary arteries, and next perhaps the legs, at the distal parts at least, where the circulation is always at a disadvantage if the patient is up and about.

SYMPTOMS

The symptoms are increased tension, which means, sooner or later, hypertrophy of the left ventricle and an accentuated closure of the aortic valve. This alone means more and more tendency to aortic irritation and aortic valve irritation, with inflammation, and later deposits of calcareous material, perhaps with stiffening of the aortic valve and narrowing, aortic stenosis being the result. If such a patient with the disease advanced to this stage must overwork, or sustains any severe muscle strain, an aneurysm of the aorta may occur. In the meantime, with the advancing degeneration of the cerebral arteries, some sudden cerebral congestion, caused by leaning over, lifting, vomiting or hard coughing, may rupture a cerebral vessel, and all the symptoms of apoplexy are present. If small hemorrhages occur in the arterioles of the extremities, of course the prognosis is not serious. Sometimes some of the smaller vessels of the brain may become obstructed and cerebral degeneration occur. If distal vessels become obstructed, as of the toes or feet, gangrene takes place unless the obstruction occurs at a place where the collateral circulation could save the part from such a death. These are some of the ultimate results of serious and final arteriosclerosis. The more frequent result, when the disease has not advanced so far, is a failing heart, either from degenerative myocarditis, coronary sclerosis or dilatation, with all the symptoms of coronary sclerosis and angina pectoris, or with the symptoms of failing circulation.

With high blood pressure to the point of beginning endarteritis, a gradually increasing force of the apex beat occurs, the aortic closure is accentuated as just described, the pulse is slow, the tensity of the arteries depends on the stage of the disease, and when the disease is actually present, the palpable arteries do not collapse on pressure. They soon lose their elasticity, and if this occurs in parts which are soft and flexible, the arteries become more or less tortuous by the force of the blood current twisting and bending them, owing to the irregularity of their hardening. The extremities readily become numb, or the part "goes to sleep," as it is termed. This occurs frequently at night. Sooner or later some edema of the feet and legs occurs in the latter part of the day. Sometimes abdominal colic attacks occur, caused by disturbed circulation. Various disturbances of metabolism may occur, depending on the circulation in the different organs or on coincident disease, and the liver, pancreas and kidneys may be affected.

The blood pressure, if taken in the arms especially, may appear excessively high, but really the actual pressure in the blood vessels may be low. This is on account of the inability to compress the hardened arteries. A heart may be weak and actually need strengthening even while the blood pressure reading is high.

The treatment of this disease is successful only in its prevention, and consists in treatment of hypertension before arteriosclerosis is present. When the disease is actually present, there is nothing to do except for the patient to stop active labor, never to overeat or overdrink, to prevent, if possible, toxemias from the bowels, to keep the colon as clean as possible, and for the physician to give the heart such medicinal aids as seem needed, vasodilators if the heart is acting too strongly, possibly small doses of cardiac tonics if the heart is acting weakly; always with the knowledge that a degenerative myocarditis may be present in considerable amount, or that coronary sclerosis may be present.

As stated above, coronary sclerosis probably seldom occurs without more general arteriosclerosis. Obstruction of the coronary arteries, however, not infrequently occurs at their orifices in conjunction with sclerosis of that region of the aorta and of the aortic valve. The more these arteries are diseased and the more they are obstructed, the more the myocardium of the heart becomes degenerated, softened and weakened, when dilatation of the ventricles, especially the left, is liable to occur. Sooner or later such a condition will cause attacks of angina pectoris and more or less pronounced symptoms of chronic myocarditis and fatty degeneration, as previously described.

TREATMENT

The treatment of a suspected coronary sclerosis is the same as that of general arteriosclerosis—primarily the elimination of anything which tends to cause high tension or to produce chronic endarteritis. When either general or local arteriosclerosis is present, the treatment which should be inaugurated comprises anything which would tend to inhibit the endarteritis and the classification—necessary periods of rest, the interdiction of all physical effort or physical strain, and the regulation of the diet, digestion and elimination. Perhaps there is no greater preventive of the advance of this disease than a diet considerably less than would be suitable for the same person when in perfect health and at his regular work. The amount of protein especially should be reduced, and the meal hours should be regular. Ordinarily all tea, coffee and tobacco should be forbidden, and alcohol should be allowed only to the aged, if allowed at all.

It has long been considered that iodin would inhibit abnormal connective tissue growth. Iodin most readily reaches the blood as sodium or potassium iodid. Large amounts of iodin are not needed to saturate the requirements of the system for iodin, from 0.1 to 0.2 gm. (1 1/2 to 3 grains) preferably of sodium iodid, twice a day, after meals given with plenty of water, being sufficient; but it should be continued in one or two doses a day not only for weeks, but for months. Whether this iodid or iodin acts per se, or acts by stimulating the thyroid gland to increased activity and therefore to more normal activity, so that it is the thyroid secretion which is of benefit, it is difficult to decide. In view of the fact that in advanced years the thyroid is always subsecreting, and after the very diseases which cause arteriosclerosis or during the diseases which cause arterinsclernsis the thyroid is generally subsecreting, it would appear that the value of iodin is in its effect in stimulating the thyroid gland.

If a small amount of thyroid secretion is evidenced by other symptoms, thyroid extract should be given. The dose need not be large, and should be small, but should be given for a considerable length of time. If the patient seems to be improving on small doses of iodid, however, and the thyroid is supposed not to be very deficient, it is better not to administer thyroid extract, unless the patient is obese.

A serum treatment given intravenously, hypodermically, by the mouth, and by the rectum was inaugurated some years ago (1901 and 1902). and is known as the "Trunecek serum." This first consisted of sodium sulphate, sodium chlorid, sodium phosphate, sodium bicarbonate and potassium sulphate in water in such amounts as to stimulate the blood plasma. Later small amounts of calcium and magnesium phosphate were added to the solution to be injected. These injections seemed to lower the blood pressure, but it is doubtful whether they have any greater ability than a proper regulation of the diet to inhibit arteriosclerosis. At any rate, these injections are but seldom used.

An important means of inhibiting disturbance from any arteriosclerosis which should be employed when possible is the climate treatment. Warm, equable climates, in which there are no sudden radical changes, are advantageous when coronary sclerosis is suspected, and warm climates are valuable in promoting the peripheral circulation and lowering the blood pressure in arteriosclerosis. These patients always require more heat than normal persons, always feel the cold severely, and their hearts always have much less disturbance, fewer irregularities and fewer attacks of pain during warm weather than during cold weather.

Simple hydrotherapeutic measures are also necessary for these patients, but baths should not be used to the point of causing debility and prostration. Applications of cold water in any form are generally inadvisable. Very hot baths are also inadvisable; but pleasantly warm baths, taken at such frequency as found to be of benefit to the individual, relax the peripheral circulation relieve the tension of the internal vessels, lessen the work of the heart, and promote healthy secretion of the skin, the skin of arteriosclerotic patients often being dry. This dry skin is especially frequent if there is any kidney insufficiency, which so soon and so readily becomes a part of the arteriosclerotic process.

If the patient is old, small doses of alcohol may act physiologically for good. In these arteriosclerotic patients the activities of alcohol should be considered from the drug point of view, not from that of all intoxicating beverage. Other drugs are considered in the discussion of hypertension.

If the heart actually fails, the treatment becomes that of chronic myocarditis and of dilatation.

Not infrequently in sclerosis of the arteries, especially of the coronary arteries, the blood pressure is not high, but low, and the heart is insufficient. In such patients cardiac tonics may be considered, but they must be used with great care. Digitalis may be needed, but it should be tried in small doses. It often makes a heart with arteriosclerosis have severe anginal attacks. On the other hand, if the heart pangs or heart aches and the sluggish circulation are due to myocardial weakness without much actual degeneration, digitalis may be of marked benefit. The value of digitalis in doubtful instances will be evidenced by an improved circulation in the extremities, a feeling of general warmth instead of chilliness and cold, an increased output of urine, and less breathlessness on slight exertion.

ANGINA PECTORIS

This is a name applied to pain in the region of the heart caused by a disturbance in the heart itself. Heart pains and heart aches from various kinds of insufficiency of the heart, or heart weakness, are not exactly what is understood by angina pectoris. It is largely an occurrence in patients beyond the age of 30, and most frequently occurs after 50, although attacks between the ages of 40 and 50 are becoming more frequent. It is a disturbance of the heart which most frequently attacks men, probably more than three fourths of all cases of this disease occurring in men; in a large majority of the cases the coronary arteries are diseased.

Various pains which are not true angina pectoris occur in the left side of the chest; these have been called pseudo-anginas. They will be referred to later. True angina pectoris probably does not occur without some serious organic disease of the heart, mostly coronary sclerosis, fatty degeneration of the heart muscle, adherent pericarditis and perhaps some nerve degenerations. Various explanations of the heart pang have been suggested, such as a spasm or cramp of the heart muscle, sudden interference with the heart's action, as adherent pericarditis, a sudden dilatation of the heart, an interference with the usual stimuli from auricle to ventricle and therefore a very irregular contraction, a sudden obstruction to the blood flow through a coronary artery, or a sudden spasm from irritation associated with some of the intercostal or more external chest muscles causing besides the pang a sense of constriction. Perhaps any one of these conditions may be a cause of the heart pang, and no one be the only cause.

In a true angina, death is frequently instantaneous. In other instances, death occurs in a few minutes or a few hours; or the patient's life may be prolonged for days, with more or less constant chest pains and frequent anginal attacks. Here there is a gradual failing of the heart muscle, with circulatory insufficiency, until the final heart pang occurs.

Anginal attacks before the age of 40, presumed, from a possible narrowing of the aortic valve, to be due to coronary sclerosis, are frequently due to a long previous attack of syphilis. In these cases, active treatment of the supposed cause should be inaugurated, including perhaps an injection of the arsenic specific, and certainly a course of mercury and iodid, with all the general measures for managing and treating general arteriosclerosis, as previously described.

SYMPTOMS

The pain of true angina pectoris generally starts in the region of the heart, radiates up around the left chest, into the shoulders, and often down the left arm. This is typical. It may not follow this course, however, but may be referred to the right chest, up into the neck, down toward the stomach, or toward the liver. The attack may be coincident with acute abdominal pain, almost simulating a gastric crisis of locomotor ataxia. There may also be coincident pains down the legs. It has been shown, as mentioned in another part of this book, that disturbances in different parts of the aorta may cause pain and the pain be referred to different regions, depending on the part affected.

Instances occasionally occur in which a patient had an anginal attack, as denoted by facial anxiety, paleness, holding of the breath, and a slow, weak pulse, without real pain. This has been called angina sine dolore. The patient has an appearanece of anxious expectation, as though he feared something terrible was about to happen.

The position of the patient with true angina pectoris is characteristic. He stops still wherever he is, stands perfectly erect or bends his body backward, raises his chin, supports himself with one hand, leans against anything that is near him, and places his other hand over his heart, although he exercises very little pressure with this hand. The position assumed is that which will give the left chest the greatest unhampered expansion, as though he would relieve all pressure on the heart.

Besides the feeling of constriction, even to some spasm, perhaps, of the intercostal muscles, respiration is slowed or very shallow, because of the reflex desire of the patient not to add to the pain by breathing. The face is pale, the eyes show fear, and the whole expression is almost typical of cardiac anxiety. The patient feels that he is about to die. The pulse is generally slowed, may be irregular, and may not be felt at the wrist. The blood pressure has been found at times to be increased. It could of course be taken only in those cases in which there were more or less continued anginal pains; the true typical acute angina pectoris attack is over, or the patient is dead, before any blood pressure determination could be made. When there is more or less constant ache or frequent slight attacks of pain, the blood pressure may be raised by the causative disease, arteriosclerosis. During the acute attack with inefficient cardiac action and a diminished force and frequency of the beat, the peripheral blood pressure can only be lowered.

The duration of an acute attack, that is, the acute pain, is generally but a few seconds, sometimes a few minutes, and rarely has lasted for several hours. In the latter cases some obstruction to an artery has been found at necropsy, but not sufficient to stop the circulation at a vital point. Repeated slight attacks, more or less severe, may occur frequently throughout one or more days, or even perhaps a series of days, caused by the least exertion, even that of turning in bed.

While most cases of sudden death with cardiac pain are due to a local disease in or around the heart, it is quite probable that some disturbance in the medulla oblongata may cause acute inhibitory stoppage of the heart through the pneumogastric (vagi) nerves. The power of the pneumogastric reflex to inhibit the action of the heart is, of course, easily demonstrated pharmacologically. Clinically reflexes down these nerves interfering with the heart's action cause faintness and serious prostration, if not actual shock, and perhaps, at times, death. The most frequent cause of such a reflex is abdominal pain, perhaps due to some serious condition in the stomach, to gastralgia, to an intestinal twist, to intussusception or other obstruction, or to hepatic or renal colic. A severe nerve injury anywhere may cause such a heart reflex. Hence serious nerve pain must always be stopped almost immediately, else cardiac and vasomotor shock will occur. In serious pain morphin becomes a life saver.

MANAGEMENT

While a number of causes of true cardiac pain may be eliminated by improvement in any loss of compensation, by improvement of the heart tone, by more or less recovery from myocardial or endocardial inflammation, and by the withdrawal of nicotin, which may cause cardiac pains, still, true angina pectoris once occurring is likely to be caused by a progressive, incurable condition, and the attacks will become more frequent until the final one. It is possible that a true angina may be due to a coronary artery disease or obstruction, and that a collateral circulation may become established and repair the deficiency. While this probably can take place, it must be rare.

Occasionally when the intense pain has ceased, the patient may be nauseated and actually vomit, or he may soon pass a large amount of urine of low specific gravity, or have a copious movement of the bowels.

The first attack, and subsequent ones more and more readily, are precipitated by any exertion which increases the work of the heart, as walking up hill, walking against the wind, going upstairs, physical strains, as suddenly getting out of bed, leaning over to put on the shoes, straining at stool, or even mental excitement. Exertion directly after eating a large meal is especially liable to precipitate an attack. Food which does not readily digest, or food which causes gastric flatulence may precipitate attacks. Any indiscretion in the use of coffee, tea, alcohol or tobacco may be the cause of the attack.

For treatment of the immediate pain, if the physician arrives soon enough, anything may be given which quickly relieves local or general arterial spasm and spasm of the muscles. The moment that the heart and its arterioles relax, the attack is often over. The most quickly acting drug for this purpose is amyl nitrite, inhaled. If amyl nitrite is not at hand, or has been found previously to cause considerable disturbance of the head or a feeling of prolonged faintness, nitroglycerin is the next most rapidly acting drug. It may be given hypodermically, or a tablet may be dissolved on the tongue. The amyl nitrite should be in the emergency case of the physician in the form of ampules, or may be carried by the patient after he has had one or more attacks. The ampules now come made of very thin glass with an absorbent and silk covering ready for crushing with the fingers, and are thus immediately ready for inhalation. One of these is generally all that it is necessary to use at any one time. Nitroglycerin, if given hypodermically, should be in dose of 1/100 grain. If given by mouth the dose should be the same, repeated in ten minutes if the pain has not stopped.

Almost coincidently with the administration of nitroglycerin or the amyl nitrite, a hypodermic injection of 1/8 or 1/6 grain of morphin sulphate should be given without atropin, as full relaxation is desired without any stimulation of atropin.

Alcohol is also a valuable treatment of this pain, when the drugs mentioned are not at hand. The dose should be large; whisky or brandy is best, and should be administered in hot or at least warm water. The physiologic action of alcohol, which dulls or benumbs the nervous system and dilates the peripheral blood vessels, is exactly in line with the clinical indications.

If a patient is home and at rest at the time of an attack, a hot- water bag but slightly filled, or a pad electrically heated, may be placed over the heart some times with marked advantage and relief from pain. Occasionally even such gentle applications are not tolerated.

After the attack is over, absolute rest for some hours, at least, is positively necessary. If the attack was severe, the patient should rest several days, as there seems to be a great tendency for such attacks to come in groups, the cause being acutely present for at least some time. But little food should be given; nothing very hot or very cold, and no large amount of liquids; gentle catharsis may be induced on the following day, if deemed advisable; no stimulating drugs should be administered, and nothing which would raise the blood pressure.

The question often arises as to whether or not the patient shall be told of the seriousness of his condition. It is hardly wise to withhold this knowledge from him, and generally is not necessary. The ordinary alert patient knows how serious the condition is by his own feelings, and will even reprove or joke with his physician for minimizing the danger. It is best that the whole subject be discussed carefully with him and his life regulated and ordered, and emergency drugs prepared and given him with proper instructions, to the family, so that he may possibly prevent other attacks and, if they occur, may have the best immediate treatment.

The acute symptoms being over, a careful analysis of the probable cause of the anginal attack should be made. If it is a general sclerosis, the treatment should be directed to that condition. If it is a myocarditis, a fatty degeneration of the heart or a fatty heart, this should be properly treated as previously described. If it is due to a toxemia from intestinal disturbance, that may readily be remedied. If due to nicotin, it need not again occur from that reason, and perhaps the damage caused by the nicotin may be removed. Any organic kidney trouble must, of course, be managed according to its seriousness, and if there is hypertension without any serious lesion, the treatment should be directed toward its relief.

Not infrequently, whether a patient is suffering from real angina pectoris or a pseudo-angina pectoris, the absorption of toxins irons the intestines, due to indigestion and fermentation, adds to these cardiac pains, and may even be a cause of them. Consequently, eliminative treatment and a temporary rigid diet, and various treatments to prevent intestinal indigestion, are of great value in angina pectoris.

It may be even advisable for twenty-four hours or so to give nothing but water, and then perhaps a skimmed milk diet for a few days. This treatment, combined with almost absolute rest, and later graded exercise, with other measures to lower the blood pressure, and with the absence of tobacco, sometimes is very successful treatment.

PSEUDO-ANGINA

While this name is more or less unfortunate, it has long been in vogue as a designation for pains and disturbances referred by a patient to his heart. Therefore with the distinct understanding that if the diagnosis is correct the name is a misnomer, it may be allowable to discuss under this heading some of the attacks which may simulate an angina and must be separated from a true angina.

To decide whether pain in the region of the heart or irregularity of its action is due to organic disease, to functional disturbance, or to referred causes is often extremely difficult. Some of the most disturbing sensations in the region of the heart are not due to any organic trouble, and yet the patient is fearful that such sensations mean some kind of heart disease, and therefore becomes exceedingly anxious and watches and mentally records every sensation in the left chest. This is unfortunate, as the patient may learn to note, if he does not actually count, his heart beats, while normally he should sense nothing of his heart's activity. On the other hand, as just stated, it may be almost impossible to decide that this disturbance of the heart is not due to an organic cause, but is entirely functional, or due to some extraneous reason.

It seems justifiable in every case of irregular heart action to assure the patient that the condition can be improved, which in most instances is the truth. There can be no question of such urgent assurance, if it is decided that the cause is not in the heart itself, or at least is not organic. Irregularities in the heart's action will be discussed later. At this time discussion will be limited to pain which is not true angina pectoris, but which is in the region of the heart or is referred to it.

Intercostal neuralgia is more likely to occur on the left side of the chest than on the right. This is particularly unfortunate, as tending to cause these pains to be referred to the heart. The localization of tender spots along the course of a nerve with demonstration of these to the patient and the diagnosis stated is all the assurance that he requires.

Careful questioning, and if necessary scientific examination of the stomach, may show that the patient has hyperchlorhydria, ulcer of the stomach or duodenum, dilatation of the stomach, or some growth in the stomach as a cause for the pain referred to the region of the heart. Gallstones in the gallbladder may also give such referred pains. Other lesions in the abdomen may cause pain referred to the cardiac region. Not only will the demonstration of these causes and their treatment assure the patient that he has not neuralgia of his heart, but also, if curable, the cause of the pain may be removed.

Dry pleurisy of the left chest is not an infrequent cause of these pains, and of course serious disease of the lungs, as tuberculosis, unresolved pneumonia, pleuritic adhesions, ennphysema and tumor growths, may all be the cause of a referred cardiac pain, the heart being disturbed secondarily.

A stomach cramp is a not infrequent cause of serious pain referred to the heart, and the rare condition of cardiospasm must also be remembered as a cause of pseudo-angina. In other words, the interpretation of these pseudo-anginas means a careful diagnosis of the condition, and, as previously stated, not only must the above-named causes be excluded, but also the reverse must be remembered: that many disturbances treated as other conditions really are due to cardiac weakness. The diagnosis of a real angina pectoris from a false angina may not be difficult. A real angina generally occurs after exertion of some kind, be that exertion ever so slight. False angina may occur at any minute with or without exertion. Pain referred to the heart which awakens a patient at night is not likely to be a true angina; nervous patients are prone to have such night attacks of cardiac disturbance of various kinds. A true angina causes the patient's face to look anxious and pale, with the breathing repressed. A false angina shows no such paleness, allows deep breathing, crying and lamenting, and allows the patient to move about in bed, or about the room. The true angina makes the patient absolutely still and quiet: he hardly dares to speak or tell what he is feeling and fearing. True angina is of course much more frequent in older persons, while false anginas occur in the young, and especially in the neurotic. With all the other manifestations of hysteria, palpitation and cardiac pain are often symptoms.

It should not be decided, however apparently self-evident that a referred pain is not due to cardiac lesion until a careful examination of the patient has been made. Real cardiac disturbance can of course occur at any time in a neurotic or hysterical patient, and there should be no mistakes of omission from carelessness or neglect on the part of the physician.

Other frequent causes of more or less disturbance of the heart's action, often accompanied by pain, are overexertion, worry and mental anxiety, and intestinal toxemias due to too much protein or disturbed protein digestion. Frequent causes are tobacco, and the overuse of tea and coffee. Many a patient's pseudo-anginas are corrected by stopping tea and coffee. The effects of caffein and tobacco on the heart will be considered later when toxic disturbances are under discussion.

The above-mentioned causes of pseudo-anginas have only to be named to indicate the treatment which will prevent the pain attacks. At times, the cause being intangible, it may be necessary to change the whole life and metabolism of the patient, as so often necessary in hysteria, neurasthenia, gout, intestinal fermentation and kidney inefficiency. Besides a rearrangement of the diet and measures for causing proper activity of the bowels, massage, exercise and hydrotherapy should lie utilized toward the end of improving the nutrition of every part.

TREATMENT OF PSEUDO-ANGINAS

The treatment of these pseudo-angibas depends, of course, on the diagnosis of the cause, and the cause should be eliminated or modified. If the heart shows real disturbance from this reflex cause, the treatment aimed toward it depends on whether the heart action is weak or strong and the circulation poor or good. If the circulation is poor, digitalis in small doses may be needed, either 5 drops of an active tincture twice a day, or 8 or 10 drops once a day. If digitalis is not indicated, strophanthus sometimes is valuable. While strophanthus has been shown not to be a real cardiac tonic like digitalis, still there seems to be a nervous sedative action when it is given by the mouth, and it often does good in these cases. The dose is 5 drops of the tincture, in water, three times a day, after meals. Strychnin in small doses may be needed, but in these patients, who are generally nervous, it is usually better not to give it.

One of the best sedatives to a heart that is irregular in its action and not acting strongly is lime; a good way to administer it is in the form of calcium lactate, and the dose is 0.3 gm. (5 grains), in powder or capsule, three times a day, after meals.

If the circulation is good and the heart is strong, and yet these irregular pains and irregular contractions occur, the bromids act favorably and successfully. This is probably on account of their ability to quiet the central nervous system, to quiet and soothe the irritability of the heart, and to relax the peripheral blood vessels. The dose should be from 0.5 to 1 gm. (7 1/2 to 15 grains), in water, three times a day, after meals. It is not necessary or advisable to continue the bromid very long. Whatever general tonic or eliminative treatment the patient, requires should be given. The value of hydrotherapy, massage and graded exercise should not be forgotten.

STOKES-ADAMS DISEASE: HEART BLOCK

Stokes-Adams disease, or the Stokes-Adams syndrome, is a name applied to a combination of symptoms which was described by Stokes in 1846, and had been observed by Adams in 1827. The disease is characterized by bradycardia and cerebral attacks, either syncope or pseudo-apoplectic or convulsive attacks.

To understand the phenomena of this disease, it will be well to refer to the first chapter of this book. Until 1893, when His described the bundle of muscle fibers which is now known by his name, the transmission of the cardiac stimulus to contraction was not understood. It has been found, by studying the pathology of Stokes-Adams disease, as well as by clinically noting with instruments the contractions of different parts of the heart, that these slow heart beats are really due to interruptions of the impulse passing from auricle to ventricle through the bundle of His, and degeneration in this region is generally the cause of Stokes- Adams disease. The auricles often beat many times more frequently than the ventricles, even two or three times as frequently, and, of course, these auricular contractions are not transmitted to the arterial system, and the radial pulse notes only the contractions of the ventricles. The phrase that is used to describe this nontransmission of the auricular stimulus to the ventricles is "heart block."

While this disease almost invariably has a pathology, cases have occurred in which no lesion of the heart could be found, but it generally occurs coincidently with arteriosclerosis, in which the coronary arteries are more or less involved and the arterial system of the brain may be diseased. It occurs more frequently in men than in women, and in them mostly after middle, or in advanced, life. The previous history of the patient has often disclosed syphilis. The intermittence of the pulse may be regular or irregular, and may not be constant in the early stages of the disease; but when the disease is established, the rate of the pulse may be reduced to forty, thirty, or even twenty beats a minute, and it has been known to be even less. When these intermittences are regular, perhaps two beats to one intermittence, or three beats to one intermittence are the most frequent types. When the auricles also beat slowly, perhaps the vagiare for some reason overstimulated and thus inhibit the heart's activity.

The attacks of syncope are doubtless due to anemia of the medulla, because of the infrequent ventricular contractions. This anemia of the medulla and of the brain may also cause an epileptic seizure, or a partial paralytic seizure without any apparent paralysis. It is probable, however, that in these cases there may be coincident arterial disease in the brain. These sudden syncopal attacks are likely to occur when a patient suddenly rises from a reclining posture, especially if he has been asleep. Many persons whose circulation is none too strong may feel faint on suddenly rising, but in a person whose pulse is slow and the circulation weak the danger of causing anemia of the brain by the sudden erect posture is much increased. Slight faint turns are of frequent occurrence with these patients; or the faintness may be so rapid and so intense that the patient may drop in his tracks. Venous pulsation in the neck is generally marked, showing an impeded contraction of tile right auricle.

If the auricles are heard or found by instrumental readings to contract more frequently than the ventricles, the trouble is quite likely to be a heart block from disease in the heart itself, in the bundle of His. If the heart is slowed as a whole, the trouble might be due to diseased arteries or pressure from a growth, a gumma, perhaps, or other brain tumor in the region of the pons Varolii or medulla oblongata; or a hemorrhage into the fourth ventricle, causing pressure, could be the cause.

TREATMENT

The treatment of true Stokes-Adams disease is unsuccessful. If general arteriosclerosis is present, that condition should be treated. Digitalis would seem almost invariably contraindicated, although it is of value in extrasystoles without heartblock, or in conditions which are not Stokes-Adams disease; but if this disease was considered present, digitalis would probably do harm. Sometimes strychnin is of benefit.

Atropin has sometimes caused stimulation of the heart to more normal rapidity. Its benefit is generally only temporary, as most patients cannot take atropin regularly without having it cause a disagreeable drying of the throat and skin, a stimulation of the brain, and an undesired raising of the blood pressure, to say nothing of its action on the eyes.

The only value of the nitrites is when the blood pressure is high and the nitrite action is desired on that account.

Coffee or caffein often causes these hearts to become irritable; it certainly raises the blood pressure, and therefore is not generally advisable. Both tea and coffee should generally be prohibited.

During the acute faint attack, camphor is one of the best stimulants. Alcohol may be of benefit. If syphilis is a cause of the condition, iodids are always valuable. If syphilis is not a cause and arteriosclerosis is present, small doses of iodid given for a long period are beneficial, although it may not much reduce the blood pressure or decrease the plasticity of the blood. Iodid is a stimulant to the thyroid gland, and therefore it is on this account valuable.

An excellent stimulant to the heart is thyroid secretion or thyroid extract. Theoretically thyroid extracts should be the treatment for a slow-acting heart. It sometimes seems of benefit to these patients, but it often causes such nervous excitation and irritability as to preclude its use. The dose of thyroid for this purpose would be small, about one-fourth to one-half grain of the active substance three times a day. To be of any value, the preparation must be good.

Epinephrin has been shown by Hirtz [Footnote: Hirtz: Arch d. mal. du coeur, February, 1916] to overcome experimental heart block. It is not clear just how it acts, but it could well be tried in heart block when the blood pressure is not too high. A few drops of an epinephrin solution 1:1,000 may be placed on the tongue, and repeated three times a day, or from 5 to 10 minims of a weaker solution may be given hypodermically.

The usual precautions against overeating, overdrinking, severe physical exercise, sudden movements, overuse of tobacco, etc., should all be urged on the patient. The disease is sooner or later fatal, although the patient may live some years. Death is generally sudden.

It is understood that this disease must he separated from the condition of bradycardia inherent in a few persons who have a slow pulse throughout their life, without any untoward symptoms.

CARDIOVASCULAR RENAL DISEASE

With the strennousness of this era, this disease or condition, which may be regarded as one of the accompaniments of normal old age, has become of grave importance, and nowadays frequently develops in early middle life. If it is diagnosed in its incipiency, and the patient follows the advice given him, the progress of the disease will generally be inhibited, and a premature old age postponed.

In the beginning the symptoms and signs of this disease are generally those of hypertension, and the treatment and management is that advised in hypertension. If the kidneys show irritation, as manifested by the presence of albumini and casts in the urine, or if they show insufficiency in the twenty-four-hour excretion of one or more salts or other excretory product, the diet and life must be more carefully regulated than advised in hypertension, and the treatment becomes practically that of chronic interstitial nephritis.

Sooner or later, in most instances of this disease, whether hypertension, chronic endarteritis or interstitial nephritis or any combination of these conditions is most in evidence, the heart will hypertrophy. As long as the circulation in the heart itself is good and not impaired by coronary sclerosis, and as long as this slowly developing chronic myocarditis has not advanced far, cardiac symptoms will not be in evidence; but if these conditions occur, or if the blood pressure is so greatly increased as to damage the aortic valve or strain and dilate the left ventricle, symptoms rapidly appear, and the heart must be carefully watched. Subsequently, as the disease advances, if the patient does not die of angina pectoris, apoplexy or uremia, the symptoms of cardiac decompensation will develop. As the heart begins to fail, a dilatation of the right ventricle causes passive congestion of the kidneys, and the chronic interstitial nephritis may progress more rapidly. It is often difficult to decide which is more in evidence, heart insufficiency or kidney insufficiency. The more the heart fails, the more albumin will generally appear in the urine, and the lower the blood pressure, especially the diastolic. The more insufficient the kidneys, the higher the blood pressure, especially the diastolic. The location of the edema will aid in deciding which condition is most in evidence. If the edema is pendent in feet, legs and perhaps genitals when the patient is up, with its disappearance at night, and more or less backache and pitting of the back in the morning, it is the heart that is most rapidly failing. If there is more general edema, the hands and face puffing, and there are considerable nausea and vomiting, headache and drowsiness, and perhaps muscular twitchings, with neuralgic pains, the most serious trouble at that particular time lies in the kidney insufficiency. Kisch [Footnote: Kisch: Med. Klin., Feb. 27, 1916.] sums up the procedural symptoms and signs of cerebral hemorrhage. The heart is generally enlarged and hypertrophied. The patient is likely to be overweight or adding weight, and to suffer from intestinal indigestions. Signs of sclerosis of the blood vessels of the brain are evidenced by transient dizziness; headaches; impaired sleep; loss of memory, especially for names and words; slight disturbances of speech, momentary perhaps, and more or less temporary localized numbness of the hands or feet, or arms or legs, with perhaps flushing of some part of the body, or little localized spasms of vessels of other parts of the body, causing chilliness.

There is also a marked hereditary tendency to apoplexy.

Cadwalader, [Footnote: Cadwalader, W. R.: A Comparison of the Onset and Character of the Apoplexy Caused by Cerebral Hemorrhage and by Vascular Occlusion, The Journal A. M. A., May 2, 1914, p. 1385.] after considerable investigation, has come to the conclusion that large hemorrhages into the brain are the rule in apoplexy, and that small hemorrhages are rare, and he is inclined to think that even small, as well as large hemorrhages, are more frequently fatal than supposed. In other words, he thinks that many of the nonfatal hemiplegias are caused by vascular obstruction and softening and not by hemorrhage. He finds that sudden death, or death within a few minutes, does not occur from hemorrhage, even if the hemorrhage is large, though a rapidly developing and persistent coma usually indicates a hemorrhage. If the coma is not profound and is slow in its onset, with symptoms noticed by the patient, and cerebral disturbance, he believes it to be caused generally by softening of the cerebral center, due to some obstruction of the blood flow, and not to hemorrhage. While occasionally a slowly increasing loss of consciousness may be due to hemorrhage, he thinks it is doubtful if real hemorrhage ever occurs without loss of consciousness, while softening of some part of the cerebrum may occur without unconsciousness. He thinks that the size of the hemorrhage is of more importance than its situation in causing the profoundness of the symptoms, but he repeats that nonfatal cases of hemiplegia are generally caused by vascular occlusion and subsequent softening, and not by hemorrhage.

TREATMENT

While it is urged, in preventing the actual development of this disease, and in slowing its progress, that it is advisable to lower a high blood pressure, we must remember that this blood pressure mad be compensatory, and many times should not be much lowered without due consideration of the symptoms and the patient's condition. It is better not to use drugs of any kind in this incipient condition. The hypertension should be regulated by the diet; the purin bases and meat should be reduced to a minimum; tea, coffee and alcohol should be prohibited, and tobacco should be either entirely stopped or reduced to a minimum. Regulated exercise is always advisable, the amount of such exercise depending on the condition of the circulation. Ordinary walking and graduated walking or graduated hill climbing and golfing are good exercise for these patients. Mental and physical strenuosity must be stopped, if the disease is to be slowed. Sleeplessness must be combated, and perhaps actually treated medicinally, and for a time sufficient doses of chloral are perhaps the best treatment. The administration of chloral must always be carefully guarded to avoid the acquirement of dependence on the drug. Mouth and other infections should be sought and removed. Warm baths, Turkish baths, electric light baths or body baking may be advisable, and certainly obesity must always be combated by a regulation of the diet. In obesity, stimulants to the appetite, such as spices, condiments, and even sometimes salt, must be prohibited. Butter, cream, sugar and starches must be reduced to a minimum. A small amount of bread and a small amount of potatoes should be allowed. Liquids with meals should be reduced. Fruits should be given freely. Intestinal indigestion should be corrected, and free daily movements of the bowels should be caused. If the patient is obese, and especially if the blood pressure is high, the administration of thyroid extract is very beneficial. This is particularly true in women suffering from this disease; but the patient should be carefully observed during its administration. It may be advisable to administer small doses of iodid instead of the thyroid treatment, or coincidently with it. Nitrites had better be postponed, if possible, for cardiac emergencies.

White, [Footnote: White: Boston Med. and Surg. Jour., Dec. 2, 1915.] after studying 200 cases of heart disease, finds that men are more subject to auricular fibrillation, auricular flutter, heart block and alternation of the pulse than are women. The greater frequency of syphilis in men than in women should be considered in this difference in frequency.

White finds that hyperthyroidism of long standing is often attended with auricular fibrillation. He does not find that alcohol, tea and coffee play much part in causing these serious disturbances of the heart. His conclusions on this subject are certainly a surprise, and do not coincide with the experience of many others. It would seem that one of the causes of the greater frequency of these disturbances in men would be the amount of alcohol and tobacco used by men.

When the heart begins to fail from a gradually progressing myocarditis, the pulse rate generally increases, especially on the least exertion, and on fast walking may be as high as 120 or 130 a minute, or even higher. It may be found near 100 on the least exertion, even after some minutes of rest. These patients must have more or less absolute bed rest. When this condition occurs in old age, however, prolonged bed rest is inadvisable, for if the heart once loses its energy, in such cases, it is practically impossible to cause a return of normal function. However, in all acute cardiac insufficiency in this disease, due to some heart strain or exertion that was unusual, a bed rest of from one to two weeks and then gradually getting up and returning to normal activity is the proper treatment, and will generally be successful in restoring more or less compensation. These patients may well recline in bed with several pillows or with a back rest. During any cardiac anxiety in this kind of insufficiency the patient breathes better when he is sitting up or reclining with the head and shoulders high. The reason for this is probably because his heart has more space in this position—the same reason that he breathes better when his stomach is empty. Very indicative of the coming cardiac insufficiency is the inability to lie at night on the left side. The pressure of the body, especially if the person is stout, interferes with the heart action and causes dyspnea and distress. Some short, fat patients with cardiac distress caused by this disease must even stand up to relieve the condition, the erect position giving still more space for the action of the heart.

Before these patients get up, after a period of bed rest, slight exercises should be done, perhaps resistant exercises, to see what the effect is on the heart, and also gradually to cause increase in cardiac strength, much as any other training exercise. Whatever exercise increases the heart rate more than twenty-five beats is too strenuous at that particular period. The exercise should then be still more carefully graduated. If the systolic blood pressure is altogether too low for the age of the person or for the previous history, it should be allowed to become higher, if possible, before much exercise is begun.

The diet should be nutritious, but, of course, modified by the condition of the stomach, intestines and kidneys, and whether or not the patient is obese. The bulk of the meal should be small, and nutriment should be given at three or four hour intervals during the daytime.

The Karell milk diet or so-called "cure" was first presented in 1865 by Phillippe Karell, physician to the Czar of Russia. This treatment was more or less forgotten until lately, when it has been more frequently used in kidney, liver and heart insufficiency. Its main object in kidney and heart disease is to remove dropsies. In cardiac dropsy it is advised to give 200 c.c. of milk for four doses at four hour intervals, beginning at 8 o'clock in the morning. Whether the milk is taken hot or cold depends on the desire of the patient. This treatment is supposed to be kept up for six days, and during this time no other fluid is given and no solid food allowed. During the next two days an egg is added to this treatment, given about 10 o'clock in the morning, and a slice of dry toast, or zwieback, at 6 p. m. Then up to the twelfth day the food is gradually increased, first to two eggs a day, then more bread, then a little chopped meat, then rice or some cereal, and by the end of two weeks the patient is about back to his ordinary diet. During this period the bowels are moved by enema or by some vegetable cathartic, or even castor oil. If thirst is excessive, the patient must have a little water, and if the desire for solid food is excessive, even Karell allowed a little white bread and at times a little salt. He sometimes even prolonged the period of treatment to five or six weeks.

Various modifications of this treatment have been suggested, such as skimmed milk, and more in quantity, or a cereal is added more or less from the beginning, and perhaps cream. The diuretic action of this treatment is not always successful. Also, sometimes the treatment is even dangerous, the heart and circulation becoming weaker than before such treatment was begun. Certainly the treatment should be used in cardiac insufficiency with a great deal of care, although it is often very valuable treatment. It should be emphasized that most patients with cardiac dropsy receiving the Karell treatment or a modification of it should also receive digitalis in full doses, and should have daily free movement of the bowels. It should be urged, however, that too free catharsis in cardiac weakness is to be avoided, and the prolonged use of salines, and sometimes even one administration is contraindicated. Before cardiac failure has occurred in this disease, once a week a dose of calomel or a brisk saline purge is advisable, and is good treatment; but when cardiac weakness has developed, free catharsis is rarely indicated, although the bowels should be daily moved, and vegetable laxatives are the best treatment. The upper intestine and the liver and kidneys may be relieved by a more or less abrupt modification of the diet, or even a starvation period, and the bowels will generally become cleaned; but frequent profuse purging with salines or some drastic cathartic puts the final touch on a cardiac failure.

Recently Goodman [Footnote: Goodman, E. H.: The Use of the "Karell Cure" in the Treatment of Cardiac, Renal and Hepatic Dropsies, Arch. Int. Med., June, 1916, p. 809.] presented a report of his studies of the Karell treatment in cardiac, renal and hepatic dropsies. He finds that patients with uremia ordinarily should not be subjected to the Karell cure, such patients needing more fluid.

As long as the patient remains in bed, and as long as his ability to exercise is at a minimum, gentle massage is advisable.

In these cases of cardiac weakness, with or without dropsy, unless the diastolic pressure is very high, digitalis is valuable. If there is no cardiac dropsy, but other symptoms of heart tire are manifest and the blood pressure is high, the nitrites are valuable. The amount should be sufficient to lower the blood pressure. Sometimes the diastolic pressure is high and the systolic low and the pressure pulse small because of heart insufficiency; such a condition is often improved by digitalis. In other words, with a failing heart digitalis may not make a blood pressure higher, and often does not; it may even lower a diastolic pressure, and the moment that the pressure pulse becomes sufficient, the patient improves. Under this treatment of digitalis, rest and regulated diet, a dilated left ventricle with a systolic mitral blow often becomes contracted and this regurgitation disappears.

The amount of digitalis that is advisable has been frequently discussed. It should be given in the best preparation obtainable, and should be pushed gradually (not suddenly) to the point of full physiologic activity. While it may be given at first three times a day in smaller doses, it later should be given but twice a day, and still later once a day, in a dose sufficient to cause the results. As soon as the full activity has been reached it may be intermitted for a short time; or it may be given a longer time in smaller dosage. In renal insufficiency associated with cardiac insufficiency, its action is subject to careful watching. If there is marked advanced interstitial nephritis, digitalis may not work satisfactorily and must be used with caution. If, on the other hand, a large part of the kidney trouble is due to the passive congestion caused by circulatory weakness, digitalis will be valuable.

In sudden cardiac insufficiency, provided digitalis has not been given in large doses a short time before, strophanthin may be given intravenously once or at most twice at twenty-four-hour intervals.

If, in this more or less serious condition of the heart weakness, there is great sleeplessness, a hypnotic must sometimes be given, and the safest hypnotic is perhaps 3 / 10 grain of morphin. One of the synthetic hypnotics, where the dose required is small, may be used a few times and even a small dose of chloral should not be feared when sleep is a necessity and large doses of synthetics are inadvisable on account of the condition of the kidneys.

The value of the Nauheim baths with sodium chlorid and carbonic acid gas still depends on the individual and the way that they are applied. If the blood pressure is low and the circulation at the periphery is poor, they bring the blood to the surface, dilating the peripheral vessels, and relieving the congestion of the inner organs and abdominal vessels, and they often will slow the pulse and the patient feels improved. If they are used warm, a high blood pressure may not be raised; if the baths are cool, the blood pressure will ordinarily be raised. Provided the patient is not greatly disturbed or exhausted by getting into and out of the bath, even a patient with cardiac dilatation may get some benefit f rom such a bath, as there is no question, in such a condition, that anything which brings the blood to the muscles and skin relieves the passive internal congestion. Sometimes these baths increase the kidney excretion. At other times these, or any tub baths, are contraindicated by the exertion and exhaustion they cause the patient; and cool Nauheim baths, or any other kind of baths, are inadvisable with high blood pressure.

DISTURBANCES OF THE HEART RATE

ARRHYTHMIA

While this terns really signifies irregularity and intermittence of the heart, it may also be broadly used to indicate a pulse which is abnormally slow or one which is abnormally fast, a rhythm which is trot correct for the age, condition and activity of the patient. Irregularity in the pulse beat as to volume, force and pressure, except such variation in the pulse wave as caused by respiration, is always abnormal. While an intermittent pulse is of course abnormal, it may be caused in certain persons by a condition which does not in the least interfere with their health and well-being.

As to whether a slow or a more or less (but not excessively) rapid pulse in any one is abnormal depends entirely on whether that speed is normal or abnormal for that person. As a general rule the heart is more rapid in women than in men. It is always more rapid in children than in adults, and generally diminishes in frequence after the age of 60, unless there is cardiac weakness or some cardiac muscle degeneration. The average frequence of the pulse in an adult who is at rest is 72 beats per minute, but a frequency of 80 is not abnormal, and a frequency of 65 in men is common; 60 is infrequent in men but normal, while up to 90 is not abnormal, especially in women, at the time the pulse is being counted.' It should always be considered that in the majority of patients the pulse is slightly increased while the physician is noting its rapidity. Anything over 90 should always be considered rapid, unless the patient is very nervous and this rapidity is considered accidental. Anything below 60 is abnormally slow. In children under 10 or 12 years of age, anything below 80 is unusual, and up to 100 is perfectly normal, at least at such time as the pulse is counted and the patient is awake.

Referring to the first chapter of this book, it will be noted that many physiologic factors must enter into the production of the normal regularity of the pulse. The stimulus must regularly begin in the auricle, must be perfectly transmitted through the bundle of His to the ventricles, the ventricles must normally contract with the normal and regular force, the valves must close normally and at the proper time, the blood pressure in the aorta must be normally constant to insure the perfect transmission of the blood to the peripheral arteries and to insure the normal circulation through the coronary arteries, and the arterioles must be normally elastic. The nervous inhibitory control through the vagi must also be normal, and there must be no abnormal reflexes of any part of the body to interfere with the normal vagus control of the heart.

While the heart beats from an inherent musculonervous mechanism, nervous interference easily upsets its normal regularity. It may be seriously slowed by nervous shock, fear or sudden peripheral contractions, spasm of muscles, or convulsive contractions, or it may be stimulated to greater rapidity by nervous excitement. It may be slowed or made rapid by reflex irritations, and it may be seriously interfered with by cerebral lesions; pressure on the vagus centers in the medulla oblongata will make it very slow. Various kinds of poisons circulating in the blood, both depressants and excitants, may affect the rapidity or the regularity of the heart. Therefore, if it is decided that a given heart is abnormally slow or abnormally rapid or is decidedly irregular or intermittent, the various causes for such interference with its normal activity must be investigated and admitted or excluded as causative factors.

Many investigations of the rhythm of children's pulses have been made, and some of the later investigations seem to show that not more than 40 percent are regular, the remaining 60 percent varying from mild irregularity to extreme irregularity.

Scientifically to determine the exact character of a pulse which is discovered by the finger on the radial artery and the stethoscope on the heart to be irregular, tracings of one or more arteries, veins and the heart should be taken. Two synchronous tracings are more accurate than one, and three of more value than two in interpreting the exact activity and regularity of the heart.

ETIOLOGY

The cause of an irregularly acting heart in an adult may be organic, as in the various forms of myocarditis, in broken compensation of valvular disease, Stokes-Adams disease, coronary disease, auricular fibrillation, auricular flutter, cerebral disease, and toxemias from various kinds of serious organic disease. The cause may be more or less functional and removable, such as tea, coffee, alcohol, tobacco, gastric indigestion and intestinal toxemia; or it may be due to functional disturbances of the heart, such as that due to what has been termed extrasystole, or to irregular ventricular contractions. A frequent cause of irregular heart action in women, more especially of increased rapidity, is hyperthyroidism.

There may be an arrhythmia due to some nervous stimulation, probably through the pneumogastric, so that the pulse varies abnormally during respiration, being accelerated during inspiration and retarded during expiration more than is normally found in adults. This condition is frequent in children, and is noticed in neurotic adults and sometimes during convalescence from a serious illness. Nervous and physical rest, with plenty of sleep and fresh, clean air so that the respiratory center is normally stiniulated, will generally improve this condition in an adult.

Extrasystoles causing arrhythmia give a more or less regularly intermittent pulse, while the examination of the heart discloses an imperfect beat or the extrasystole which is not transmitted or acted on by the ventricles, and hence the intermittency in the peripheral arteries. This condition may be due to some toxemia, nervous irritability, or some irritation in the heart muscle. Good general elimination by catharsis, warm baths to increase the peripheral circulation, a low diet for a few days, abstinence from any toxin which could cause this cardiac irritation, extra physical and mental rest, sometimes nervous sedatives such as bromids, and perhaps a lowering of the blood pressure by nitroglycerin, if such is indicated, or an increase of the cardiac tone by digitalis if that is indicated, will generally remove the cardiac irritation and prevent the extrasystoles, and the heart will again become regular. It should be carefully decided whether there is beginning heart block or beginning Stokes-Adams disease, in which case digitalis should not be used. This disease is not frequent, while extrasystoles of a functional character are very frequent. Sometimes this functional disease persists without any apparent injury to the individual as long as the ventricle does not take note of these extra auricular systoles and does not also become extra rapid. If the ventricle does contract with this increased rapidity, it soon wears itself out, and the condition becomes serious.

In this kind of arrhythmia, if there are no contraindications to digitalis, it is the logical drug to use from its physiologic activities, slowing the heart by its action on the vagi and causing a steadier contraction of the heart; clinically this treatment is generally successful. If digitalis should, however, cause the heart to become more irritable, it is acting for harm, and should be stopped.

TREATMENT

One has but to refer to the enumerated causes of irregular heart action to determine the treatment. In that caused by extrasystole, the treatment has just been suggested. In irregular heart caused by serious cardiac or other lesions the treatment has already been described, or is that of the disease that has a badly acting heart as a complication. If the irregularity is caused by toxins, the treatment is to stop the ingestion of the toxin and to promote the elimination of what is already in the system; how much of the irregularity was due to the toxin and how much is inherent disturbance in the heart can then be determined. If the cause of a toxemia developed in the system, perhaps most frequently from intestinal putrefaction, increased elimination and a regulation of the diet will cure the condition.

The valvular lesions most apt to cause irregular action of the heart are mitral insufficiency or mitral stenosis. The lesion which is most apt to cause auricular fibrillation and more or less permanently irregular heart is perhaps mitral stenosis. Another frequent cause of more or less permanent irregularity is the excessive use of alcohol.

While an irregular pulse and an irregular heart are always of more or less serious import, still, as the extrasystoles of the auricle are better understood and more frequently recognized, and the habits and life of the patients (most frequently men) are regulated and revised, frequently a pulse and heart which would be rejected by any medical examiner for an insurance company becomes, in a few weeks or a few months, a perfectly acting heart, and remains so sometimes for years. It also is not quite determinaible whether a heart that is so misbehaving has a recurrence of such misbehavior more readily than a heart which has never been so affected. However this may be, the cause having been determined or presumed by the physician, it should be so impressed on the patient that he does not again repeat the insult to his heart.

AURICULAR FIBRILLATION: AURICULAR FLUTTER

Auricular fibrillation is at times apparently a clinical entity much as is angina pectoris, but it is often a symptom of some other condition. At times auricular fibrillation is only a passing symptom, and is rapidly cured by treatment. A real auricular fibrillation shows a semiparalysis of the auricles, and during this condition normal systolic contractions do not occur, although there are small rapid twitchings of different muscle fibers in the auricles. Although it was once thought that the auricle was paralyzed in this condition, it probably simply loses its coordinate activity. Auricular fibrillation and auricular flutter are probably simply different degrees of the same condition, and any contractions of the auricles over 200 per minute may be termed an auricular flutter, and below that the term auricular fibrillation may be used. When ventricular fibrillation occurs, the condition is serious and the prognosis bad. Both auricular fibrillation and auricular flutter may be temporary or permanent, and the exact number of fibrillations or tremblings of the auricular muscle can be noted only by electrical instruments.

Tallman, [Footnote: Tallman: Northwest Med., May, 1916] after examination of fifty-eight cases, classifies different types of auricular flutter: (1) such a condition in an apparently normal heart; (2) the condition occurring during chronic heart disease, and (3) an auricular flutter with partial or complete heart block.

The irregular pulse in auricular fibrillation is more or less distinctive, being generally rapid, from 110 upward. Occasionally the pulse rate may be much slower, if the heart is under the influence of digitalis. The irregularity of the pulse in this condition is excessive; the rate, strength and apparent intermittency during a half minute may not at all represent the condition in the next half minute, or in the next several minutes. If digitalis does not cure the irregularity, the condition has been termed the "absolutely irregular heart." Other terms applied to the condition have been "ventricular rhythm," "nodal rhythm" and "rhythm of auricular paralysis." The condition of the pulse has been Latinized as pulsus irregularis perpetuus.

While the condition is best diagnosed by tracings taken simultaneously of the apex beat, jugular and radial, still the jugular tracing is almost conclusive in the absence of the auricular systolic wave. The radial tracing is exceedingly suggestive, and if there is also a careful auscultation of the heart, a presumptive diagnosis may be made.

OCCURRENCE

This condition of auricular fibrillation occurs occasionally in valvular disease, and perhaps most frequently in mitral stenosis; but it can occur without valvular lesions, and with any valvular lesion. If it occurs in younger patients, valvular disease is apt to be a cause; if in older patients, sclerosis or myocardial degeneration is generally present.

It may also follow infections such as diphtheria, or some infection which has caused a myocarditis. Rarely this fibrillation may be caused by some of the drugs used to stimulate the heart.

It is astonishing how few symptoms may be present with auricular fibrillation and an absolutely irregular heart action. The patient may be able to perform all of his duties, however strenuous, until coincident, concomitant or causative ventricular weakening and dilatation of the ventricles or broken compensation occurs, and then the symptoms are those due to the cardiac failure. Often in the first stage of this weakening and later fibrillation of the auricles the patient may recognize the cardiac irregularity and disturbances. Generally, however, he soon becomes accustomed to the sensations, and, unless he has cardiac pains or dyspnea, he becomes oblivious to the irregularity. At other times he may be conscious of irregular, strong throbs or pulsations of the heart, as such hearts often give an occasional extra sturdy ventricular contraction. These he notes. Real attacks of tachycardia may be superimposed on the condition. Sooner or later, however, if the condition is not stopped, cardiac weakness and decompensation, with all the usual symptoms, occur. It seems to be probable that more than half of all cases of heart failure are due to auricular fibrillation, or at least are aggravated by it.

As previously stated, ventricular fibrillation is a very serious condition, and may be a cause of sudden death in angina pectoris, and is probably then caused by disturbed circulation in one of the coronary arteries causing an irregular blood supply to one or other of the ventricles. Absorption of some toxins or poisons which could act on the blood supply of the ventricles could also be a cause of this condition. This irregular ventricular contraction sometimes displaces the apex beat.

PATHOLOGY

Schoenberg [Footnote: Schoenberg: Frankfurt. Ztschr. f. Pathol., 1909, ii, 4.] finds that in auricular fibrillation there are definite signs in the node, such as round cell infiltration, showing inflammation, a fibrosis of the tissue, and perhaps a sclerosis of the blood vessels of that region. He also found that compression of this nodal region of the auricle from some growth or other disturbance in the mediastinal region could cause auricular fibrillation.

Jarisch [Footnote: Jarisch: Deutsch. Arch. f. klin. Med., 1914, cxv, 376.] finds by personal investigations and by studying the literature that the node showed pathologic disturbance in less than half the cases. Consequently, although a pathologic condition of the node is a frequent, and perhaps the most frequent, cause of auricular fibrillation, other conditions, especially anything which dilates the right auricle, may cause it.

DIAGNOSIS

If the pulse is intermittent and there is apparently a heart block. Stokes-Adams disease should be considered as possibly present, and digitalis would be contraindicated and would do harm.

A scientific indication as to whether a heart is disturbed through the action of the vagi or whether the disturbance is due to muscle degeneration may be obtained by the administration of atropin. Talley [Footnote: Talley, James: Am. Jour. Med. Sc., October, 1912.] of Philadelphia shows the diagnostic value of this drug. It is a familiar physiologic fact that stimulation of the vagi slows the heart or even stops it. Stimulation of these nerves by the electric current, however, does not destroy the irritability of the heart; indeed, the heart may act by local stimulation after it has been stopped by pneumogastric stimulation. It is also a well known fact that anything which inhibits or removes vagus control of the heart allows the heart to become more rapid, since these nerves act as a governor to the heart's contractions. Under the influence of atropin the heart rate is increased by paralysis of the vagi. Talley states that a hypodermic injection of from 1/50 to 1/25 grain of atropin produces the same paralytic and rapid heart effect in man. He advises the use of 1/25 grain of atropin in robust males, and 1/50 grain in females and in less robust males, and he has seen no serious trouble occur from such injections. The throat is of course dry, and the eyesight interfered with for a day or more, but Talley has not seen even insomnia occur, to say nothing of nervous excitation or delirium. Theoretically, however, before such atropin dosage, an idiosyncrasy against belladonna should be determined.

The value of such an injection rests on the fact that atropin thus injected will increase the normal heart from thirty to forty beats a minute, and Talley believes that if the heart beat is increased only twenty or less, if the patient has not been suffering from an exhausting disease, it shows "a degenerative process in the cardiac tissue which makes the outlook for improvement under treatment unpromising." He also believes that when the heart in auricular fibrillation is increased the normal amount or more than normal, the prognosis is good. He still further advises in auricular fibrillation an injection of atropin before digitalis has been administered, and another after digitalis is thoroughly acting. Comparison of the findings after these two injections will determine which factor, vagal or cardiac tissue, is the greater in the condition present. The patients with a large cardiac factor are the ones who may be more improved by the digitalis treatment than those in whom the fibrillation is caused by vagus disturbance.

PROGNOSIS

The prognosis depends on the condition of the myocardium of the vagus. If this muscle is intact, and there is no pathologic condition in the sinus node (which can be proved by the successful results of treatment), the removal of all toxins that could increase the activity of the heart, and the administration of digitalis, which will slow the heart by stimulating the pneumogastric control of the heart, will produce a cure, temporary, if not permanent.

Although a patient with auricular fibrillation may have been incapacitated by this heart activity, he may not yet have dilated ventricles, and the digitalis need perhaps not be long continued. If on account of some heart strain or some unaccountable cause the fibrillation recurs, he of course must again receive the digitalis. If the auricular fibrillation is superimposed, or is followed by dilated ventricles and decompensation, the prognosis is bad, although the condition may be improved. In other words, auricular fibrillation added to these conditions is serious, but still, many times a patient may be greatly improved by rest, digitalis, careful diet, proper care of the bowels, etc. If the fibrillation occurs with or was apparently caused by the dilatation of the ventricles, the prognosis of improvement may be good. If the dilatation of the ventricles occurs following auricular fibrillation, the prognosis is not good.

White [Footnote: White: Boston Med. and Surg. Jour., Dec. 2, 1915.] after studying 200 heart cases, finds that auricular fibrillation and alternating pulse, as well as heart block, are more frequent in men than in women, and both auricular fibrillation and alternating pulse are more apt to occur after 50 years of age than before. Auricular fibrillation may occur in hearts which are suffering from valvular lesions, especially mitral stenosis, and may occur in syphilitic hearts, in various sclerotic conditions of the heart, and in hyperthyroidism.

Though disputed, it seems probable that fibrillation may be caused by the excessive use of tea, coffee and tobacco. Paroxysmal tachycardias are certainly caused by these substances, and the conditions of auricular fibrillation and auricular flutter may be found frequently present if such hearts are carefully examined with cardiographic instruments.

TREATMENT

The condition may be stopped by relieving the heart and circulation of all possible toxins and irritants, and by the administration of digitalis. One attack is frequently followed by others, perhaps of longer duration. Occasionally, however, the patient may be observed for many years without the condition again being present. If the pulse, in spite of treatment, is permanently irregular, and auricular insufficiency is permanent, the patient is of course in danger of cardiac failure; but still he may live for years and die of some other cause than heart failure. The prognosis is better when the pulse is not rapid—below a hundred. This shows that the ventricles are not much excited and do not tend to wear themselves out.

Any treatment which lowers the heart rate is of advantage, such as the stopping of tea and coffee, and the administration of digitalis, together with rest and quiet.

While large doses of digitalis are advised, and large doses are given as soon as a patient with auricular fibrillation comes under treatment, such large dosage is dangerous practice. Many patients may be cured or may survive fluidram doses of the official tincture, but such large doses should never be used unless it is decided, after consultation, that, though dangerous, it may be a life-saving treatment.

If a patient has not been receiving digitalis, it is best to begin with a small close and gradually increase the dosage, rather than to give the heart a sudden shock from an enormous dose of digitalis. The preparation selected must be the best obtainable, but the exact dosage of any preparation can be determined only by its effect, as all preparations of digitalis deteriorate sooner or later. It is well to administer digitalis at first three times a day, then as soon as its action is thoroughly established, reduce to twice a day, and later to once a day, in such dosage as is needed to make a profound impression on the heart. The first dose may be from 5 to 10 drops, and the dosage may be increased by 5 drops at each dose, until improvement is obtained. If the patient is in a momentary serious condition and liable to die of heart failure, it is doubtful if digitalis pushed at that time will be of benefit. On the other hand, if, after consultation, it is deemed advisable to give half a fluidram or more of digitalis at once, it is justifiable. It should be emphasized that the proper dose of digitalis is enough to do the work. If within a few days there is no marked improvement, the prognosis is not good. Also, if the digitalis causes cardiac pain when such was not present, or increases cardiac pains already in evidence, and causes a tight feeling in the chest, nausea or vomiting, or a diminished amount of urine, and a tight, bandlike feeling in the head, digitalis is not acting well, and should be stopped, or the dose is too large. Also, if there is kidney insufficiency, or if the digitalis diminishes the output of urine, it generally should be stopped.

If the blood pressure is high, and perhaps almost always, even in those who are accustomed to the use of it, tobacco should be stopped. Tea and coffee should always be withheld from such patients.

The food and drink should be small in amount, frequently given, and should be such as especially to meet the needs of the individual, depending entirely on his general condition and the condition of his kidneys.

PULSUS ALTERNANS

By this term is meant that condition of pulse in which, though the rhythm is normal, strong and weak pulsations alternate. White [Footnote: White: Am. Jour. Med. Sc., July, 1915, p. 82.] has shown that this condition is not infrequent, as demonstrated by polygraphic tracings. He found such a condition present In seventy- one out of 300 patients examined, and he believes that if every decompensating heart with arrhythmia was graphically examined, this condition would be frequently found. The alternation may be constant, or it may occur in phases. It is due to a diminished contractile power of the heart when the heart muscle has become weakened and a more or less rapid heart action is present.

Gordinier [Footnote: Gordinier: Am. Jour. Med. Sc., February, 1915, p. 174.] finds that most of these patients with alternating pulse are suffering from general arteriosclerosis, hypertension, chronic myocarditis, and chronic nephritis, in other words, with cardiovascularrenal disease. He finds that it frequently occurs with Cheyne-Stokes respiration, and continues until death. He also finds that the condition is not uncommon in dilated hearts, especially in mitral disease, and with other symptoms of decompensation.

White found that about half of his cases of pulsus alternans showed an increased blood pressure of 160 mm. or more; 62 percent. were in patients over 50 years of age, and 69 percent. were in men. Necropsics on patients who died of this condition showed coronary sclerosis and arteriosclerotic kidneys.

The onset of dyspnea, with a rapid pulse, should lead one to suspect pulsus alternans when such a condition occurs in a person over 50 with cardiovascular-renal disease, arid with signs of decompensation, and also when such a condition occurs with a patient who has a history of angina pectoris.

While the forcefulness of the varying beats of an alternating pulse may be measured by blood pressure instruments by the auscultatory method, White and Lunt [Footnote: White, P. D. and Lunt, L. K.: The Detection of Pulsus Alternans, THE JOURNAL A. M. A., April 29, 1916, p. 1383.] find that in only about 30 percent. of the cases, the graver types of the condition, is this a practical procedure.

Pulsus alternans, except when it is very temporary, Gordinier finds to be of grave import, as it shows myocardial degeneration, and most patients will die from cardiac insufficiency in less than three years from the onset of the disturbance.

The treatment is rest in bed and digitalis, but White found that in only four patients out of fifty-three so treated was the alternating pulse either "diminished or banished." In a word, the only treatment is that of decompensation and a dilated heart, and when such a condition occurs and is not immediately improved, the prognosis is bad, under any treatment.

BRADYCARDIA

The first decision to be made is what constitutes a slow pulse or slow heart. A pulse below 58 or 60 beats per minute should be considered slow, and anything below 50 should be considered abnormally slow and a condition more or less suspicious. A pulse from 45 to 50 per minute occasionally occurs when no pathologic excuse can be found, but such a slow rate is unusual. Before determining that the heart is slow, it must of course be carefully examined to determine if there are beats which are not transmitted to the wrist; also whether a slow radial rate is not due to intermitence or a heart block. Auricular fibrillation, while generally causing a rapid pulse (though by no means all beats are transmitted to the peripheral arteries), tray cause a slow pulse because some of the contractions of the heart are not transmitted.

While any pulse rate below 50 should be considered abnormal and more or less pathologic, still a pulse rate no lower than 60 may, be very abnormal for the individual. For athletes and those who work hard physically, a slow pulse is normal. Such hearts are often not even normally stimulated by high fever, so that the pulse is unusually slow, considering the patient's temperature, unless inflammation of the heart has occurred.

Some chronic diseases cause a slow pulse; this is especially true of chronic interstitial nephritis. In fact, it may be stated that any disease or condition which increases the blood pressure generally slows the pulse, unless the heart itself is affected. This is true of hypertension, of arteriosclerosis, of nicotin unless the heart has become injured, and often of caffein, unless it acts in the individual as a nervous stimulant. Chronic lead poisoning causes a slow pulse on account of the increased blood pressure.

A slow pulse may occur during convalescence from acute infections, such as typhoid fever and pneumonia, and sometimes after septic processes. While it may not be serious in these conditions, it should always be carefully watched, as it may show a serious myocarditis.

While weakness generally and myocarditis, at least oil exertion or nervous excitation or after eating, cause a heart to be rapid, still such a heart may act sluggishly when the patient is at rest, so that he feels faint and weak and disinclined to attempt even the slightest exertion. In such a condition calcium, iron and strychnin, not too frequently or in too large doses, and perhaps caffein, are indicated. Camphor is always a valuable stimulant, more or less frequently administered, during such a period of slow heart. This slow heart sometimes occurs after rheumatic fever; it is quite frequent after diphtheria, and may show a disturbance of the vagi.

Although the prognosis of such slow hearts after serious illness is generally good, a heart that is too rapid after illness is often more readily brought to normal by proper management than a heart which is too slow. Either condition needs proper treatment and proper management.

It is well recognized that serious, almost major hysteria may be present and the heart not only not be increased, but it may even be slowed. The heart in this condition of course requires no treatment. In cerebral disturbances, especially when there is cerebral pressure, and more particularly if there is pressure in the fourth ventricle, the pulse may be much slowed. It is often slowed in connection with Cheyne-Stokes respiration. It may be very slow after apoplexy, and when there are brain tumors. It is often much slowed in narcotic poisoning, especially in opium, chloral and bromid poisoning. Serious toxemia from alcohol may cause a heart to be very slow. It is more likely, however, to cause a heart to be rapid, unless there is actual coma.

A frequent condition causing a slowing of the heart is the presence of bile in the blood, typically true of catarrhal jaundice. Uremic poisoning and acidemia and coma of diabetes tray cause a pulse to be very slow.

Not infrequently after parturition the heart quiets down from its exertion to a rate below normal. If the urine is known to be free from albumin and casts, and there are no signs of impending eclampsia, the slow pulse is indicative of no serious trouble; but the urine should be carefully examined and a possible uremia or other cause of eclampsia carefully considered. Sometimes with serious edema and after serious hemorrhage the heart becomes very slow, unless some exertion is made, when it will beat more rapidly than normal. This probably represents a diminished cardiac nutrition.

The cardiac lesions which cause a pulse to be slow are sclerosis or thrombosis of the coronary arteries, fatty degeneration of the myocardium, and Stokes-Adams disease.

It is seen, therefore, that when a pulse is slower than normal, even below 65 beats per minute, the cause should be sought. If no functional or pathologic excuse is discovered, it must be considered normal, for the individual, and, as stated above, even 58 or 60 beats per minute are in many instances normal for men. This is especially true with beginning hypertension, and may be true in young men who are athletic or who are oversmoking but are not being poisoned by the nicotin, as shown by the fact that their hearts are not rapid, that they are not having cardiac pains, that they do not perspire profusely, and that they do not have muscle cramps. A pulse of from 50 to 55 is likely to be seriously considered by an insurance company in deciding the advisability of the risk, and below 50 must be considered as abnormal.

SYMPTOMS

If a person has been long accustomed to a slow-acting heart, there are no symptoms. If the heart has become slowed from disease or from any acute condition, the patient is likely to feel more or less faint, perhaps have some dizzines, and often headache, which is generally relieved by lying down. Sometimes convulsions may occur, epileptiform in character, due possibly to anemia or irritation of the brain. If the slow heart does not cause these more serious symptoms, the patient may feel week and unable to attend to his ordinary duties. As previously urged an abnormally slow heart after serious illness should be as carefully cared for as a too rapid heart under the same conditions. Probably often a myocarditis and perhaps some fatty degeneration are at the base of such a slowed heart after serious infections.

A heart which has not always been slow but has gradually become slow with the progress of hypertension and arteriosclerosis will often disclose on postmortem examination serious lesions of the coronary arteries.

Deficiency in the thyroid secretion will always cause a heart to be slower than normal. The more marked and serious the hypothyroidism, the slower the heart is apt to be. When such a condition is diagnosed, the treatment is thyroid extract; or if the insufficiency is not great, small doses of an iodid should be given. In either case it is sometimes astonishing how rapidly a slow, sluggishly acting heart, improves and how much improvement there is in the mental condition of the patient.

In acute slowing of the heart, as in syncope, the patient must immediately lie down with the head low, possibly with the feet and legs elevated, and all constricting clothing of the abdomen and chest should be removed. Whiffs of smelling-salts may be given; whisky, brandy or other quickly acting stimulant, not much diluted, play also be given. Camphor, a hypodermic dose of strychnin or atropin if deemed necessary, a hot-water bag over the heart, and massaging of the arms and legs to aid the return circulation, are all means which are generally successful in restoring the patient's circulation to normal. Caffein is another valuable stimulant, perhaps best administered as a cup of coffee. Digitalis is not indicated: neither is nitroglycerin, unless the slow heart is due to cardiac pain or to angina.

Some patients have syncopal attacks with the least injury or with any mental shock. Such patients as soon as restored are as well as ever. Other patients who faint or have attacks of syncope should remain at rest on a couch or bed for some hours.

A tangible cause, being discovered for an unusually slow heart is sufficiently indicative of the treatment not to require further comment. While generally toxins from intestinal indigestion make a heart irritable and more rapid, sometimes they slow a heart, and in such cases the heart will be improved when catharsis has been caused and a modification of the diet is ordered.

PAROXYSMAL TACHYCARDIA

This condition is generally termed by the patient a "palpitation," and palpitation of the heart is recognized by most physicians as meaning a too rapidly acting heart, the term "tachycardia" being reserved for an excessive rapidity of the heart. Many of the so- called tachycardias are really instances of auricular fibrillation or flutter. Some persons normally have a pulse and heart too rapid; children more or less constantly have a heart beat of from 90 to 100. Women have more rapid heart action than men, and it becomes more rapid with their varying functions, specifically increasing its rapidity before, and perhaps during, menstruation. Many patients have a rapid heart action with the slightest increase in temperature and in any fever process. Some have a rapid heart action after the least exertion without any cardiac lesion or assignable excuse for such rapidity. Others have a rapid heart with mental activity and excessive excitement. Therefore in deciding that a heart is abnormally rapid one must individualize the patient.

During or after illness many patients are said to have palpitation when the real cause is an unhealed myocarditis. Tuberculosis almost invariably causes increased heart action, even when there is no fever. All high fever increases the heart's action, but not so markedly in typhoid fever as in other fevers; in fact, the heart in typhoid fever, during the early stages, is apt to be slower than the temperature would seem to call for. In anemia when the patient is active the heart is generally rapid. The rapid heart from cardiac disease has already been considered. For the palpitation or rapid heart Just described there is little necessity for other treatment than what the acute or chronic condition would call for. With proper management the condition will improve unless the patient has an idiosyncrasy for intermittent attacks of slightly rapid heart, as from 100 to 120 beats per minute.

A permanently rapid heart, when the patient has no heart lesion and is at rest, is generally due to hypersecretion of the thyroid, which will be discussed later. Paroxysmal tachycardia is a name applied to very rapid heart attacks in persons who are more or less subject to their recurrence. They may occur without any tangible excuse, and are liable to occur during serious illness, after a large meal, after a cup of tea or coffee, or after taking alcohol. The heart may beat as rapidly as from 150 to 200 times a minute, or even more, with no other symptoms than a feeling of constriction or tightness in the chest, an inability to respire properly and a feeling of "air hunger." The patient almost invariably must sit up, or at least have his head raised. Attacks of cardiac delirium (often auricular fibrillation) may occur with serious lesions of the heart, as valvular disease or sclerosis, but paroxysmal tachvcardia occurs in certain persons without any tangible cardiac excuse. The auricles of the heart may act more energetically than normal, and precede as usual the ventricular contraction; or the auricles and ventricles may contract almost together—a so-called "nodal" type of contraction. Rarely does a patient die of paroxysmal tachycardia. The length of time the attack may last varies from a few minutes to an hour, or even for a day or more.

MANAGEMENT

There is no specific treatment for paroxysmal tachycardia. What is of value in one patient may be of no value in another; in fact, drugs are rarely successful in ameliorating or preventing the condition. Patients who are accustomed to these attacks often learn what particular position or management stops the attack.

Sometimes a patient rises and walks about. Sometimes an ice-bag over the heart will stop the attack.

If there is no serious illness present, and no serious cardiac disease causing the condition, and a patient is known to have an overloaded stomach or bowels, an emetic or a briskly acting cathartic is the best possible treatment. The attack often terminates as suddenly as it begins, without leaving any knowledge as to which particular treatment has been beneficial. A patient who is well and has an attack of tachycardia should be allowed to assume the position which he finds to give him the most comfort, and to use the means of stopping his attack which lie has found the most successful. In the absence of his success or of his knowledge of any successful treatment, a hypodermic injection of 1/6 or even 1/4 grain of morphin sulphate is often curative. Atropin should not be given, as it may increase the cardiac disturbance. If an attack lasts more than an hour or so, one of the best treatments is the bromids, which should be given either by potassium or sodium bromid in a dose of 2 or 3 gm. (30 or 45 grains) at once. Sometimes one good-sized dose of digitalis may be of benefit, but it is often disappointing, and unless there is a valvular lesion with signs of broken compensation, it is rarely indicated. It should also be remembered that, if the patient is receiving digitalis in good dosage for broken compensation, tachycardia may be caused by an overaction of the digitalis. Such overaction would be indicated by previous symptoms of nausea, vomiting, intestinal irritation, a diminished amount of urine, headache and a tight, bandlike feeling in the head, cold hands and feet, and a day or two of very slow pulse. If none of these symptoms is present, though a patient has received digitalis for broken compensation, a tachycardia occurring might not contraindicate digitalis, as much of the digitalis on the market is useless; and a patient may not actually have been obtaining digitalis action.

If the tachycardia occurs in a patient with arteriosclerosis, especially if there is much cardiac pain, nitroglycerin is of advantage; also warm foot-baths. If there is prostration and a flaccid, flabby abdomen, a tight abdominal bandage may be of benefit.

Gastric flatulence, while perhaps not a cause of the tachycardia, is liable to develop and be a troublesome symptom. Anything that causes eructations of gases is of benefit, as spirit of peppermint, aromatic spirit of ammonia or plain hot water. If there is hyperacidity of the stomach, sodium bicarbonate or milk of magnesia will be of benefit.

The ability of some patients to stand a rapid heart action without noting it or being incapacitated by it is astonishing. It may generally be stated that a rapid heart is noted, and a pulse above 120 generally prostrates, at least temporarily, a patient who is otherwise well, provided the cause is anything but hyperthyroidism. A patient who has hypersecretion of the thyroid will be perfectly calm, collected, often perhaps not seriously nervous, and, with a heart beating at the rate of 140, 150, 160 and even 200 per minute, will state that she has no palpitation now, although she sometimes has it. A heart thus fast, with a patient not noting it and not prostrated by it, is almost diagnostic of a thyroid cause.

Some patients, both men and women, cannot take even a small cup of tea or coffee without an attack of paroxysmal tachycardia. Such patients, of course, quickly learn their limitations.

HYPERTHYROIDISM

The presence of a well marked case of exophthalmic goiter is not necessary for the secretion of the thyroid to be increased sufficiently to cause tachycardia; in fact, an increased heart rapidity in women often has hyperthyroidism as its cause. The thyroid gland hypersecretes in women before every menstrual period and during each pregnancy, and with an active, emotional, nervous life, social excitement, theaters, too much coffee, and, unfortunately today among women, too much alcohol, it readily gives the condition of increased secretion; and the organ that notes this increased secretion the quickest is the heart.

The tachycardia of a developed exophthalmic goiter is difficult to inhibit. Digitalis is of no avail, and no other single medicinal treatment is of any great value. The tachycardia will improve as the disease improves. On the other hand, nothing is snore serious for this patient than her rapid heart, and if it cannot be soon slowed, operative interference is absolutely necessary. If the rapid heart continues until a myocarditis has developed and a weakening of the muscle fibers occurs, or dilatation is imminent or has actually occurred, operative interference is serious, and most patients under these conditions die after a complete operation, that is, the removal of from one half to two thirds of the thyroid. In such cases the only excusable operative interference is the graded one, namely, the tying of first one artery and then another of the thyroid to inhibit the blood supply to the gland in order that it may not furnish so much secretion. If the heart then improves, a more radical operation may be done without much serious danger. Therefore the working rule should be that, if a heart does not quickly improve under medical management, operative interference should not be delayed until the heart has become degenerated.

If tachycardia is the only serious symptom present in a patient who is considered to have hyperthyroidism, it may generally be successfully treated by insistence on quiet, cessation of all physical and exciting mental activities, more or less complete rest, the absolute interdiction of all tear coffee or other caffein- bearing preparations, total abstinence from alcohol, the restriction to a cereal and fruit diet (the withdrawal of all meat from the diet), the administration of calcium, as the calcium glycerophospate in dose of 0.3 gm. (5 grains) in powder three times a day, and for a time, perhaps, the administration of bromids. If the depressing action of bromids on the heart is counteracted by the coincident administration of digitalis, they will act only for good by quieting the nervous system and more or less inhibiting the secretion of the thyroid gland.

If a patient has exophthalmic goiter fully developed, absolute rest in bed, with the treatment outlined above, should soon cause improvement. If it does not, the operative treatment as advised above should be considered. If myocarditis has been diagnosed, the minor operations should be done if the patient does not soon improve. The prolongation of the treatment depends on the condition and the amount of improvement.

If the physician is in doubt as to whether or not this particular tachycardia is caused by hyperthyroidism, the administration of sodium iodid in doses of 0.25 gm. (4 grains) three times a day will make the diagnosis positive within a few days. If the trouble is due to hyperthyroidism, all of the symptoms will be aggravated; there will be more palpitation, more nervousness, more restlessness, more sweating and more sleeplessness. In such cases the iodid should be stopped immediately, of course, and the proper treatment begun.

TOXIC DISTURBANCES AND HEART RATE

Under this head it is not proposed to consider disturbances of the heart due to infections, to cardiac disease, or to localized or general acute or chronic disease, but to discuss disturbances due to the absorption of irritants froth the intestines, and to alcohol, tobacco and caffein.

It is hardly necessary to repeat that various toxins which may seriously irritate the heart may be absorbed from the intestines during fermentation or putrefactives processes in either the small or the large intestines. The heart may be slowed by some, made rapid by others, and it is often made irregular. The relation of the absorption of intestinal toxins to increased blood pressure has already been described, and the necessity of removing from the diet anything which perpetuates or increases intestinal indigestion in all cases of high blood pressure has already been referred to several times. The indications that such a condition of the intestines is present are irregular action of the bowels, a large amount of intestinal gas, sometimes watery stools, often a coated tongue, and the presence of indican in the urine.

INTESTINAL PUTREFACTION

The most successful procedure in the management of intestinal putrefaction is to remove meat from the diet absolutely. Laxatives in some form are generally indicated, and one of tile best is agar- agar. Of course aloin and cascara are always good laxatives, with an occasional dose of calomel or saline, if such seem indicated. Some of the solid hydrogen peroxid-carrying preparations (magnesium peroxid, calcium peroxide [Footnote: See N. N. R., 1916, p. 232]) have been advised as bowel antiseptics, but they are not more successful than many of the salicylic acid preparations,' and perhaps none is more efficient than salol (phenyl salicylate) in a dose of 0.3 gm. (5 grains), three or four times a day. Washing out the colon with high injections is often of great value, but should not be continued too long lest the rectum become habituated to distention, and bowel movements not take place without an enema.

Lactic acid bacilli, best the Bulgarian, arc often of value in intestinal fermentation. A tablet may be eaten with a little lactose or a small lump of sucrose after each meal. Or yeast may be taken in the forth of brewer's yeast, a tablespoonful in a glass of water, two or three times a day, or one sixth of an ordinary compressed yeast cake dissolved is a glass of `eater and taken once or twice a day. Or various forms of lactic acid fermented milk may be successful.

Any particular food which causes fermentation in the intestine of the patient should be eliminated from his diet; the patient must be individualized as to fruits, cereals and vegetables, Nit, as stated above, meat should ordinarily be withheld for a time at least.

ALCOHOL

Enough has already been said of the value and limitations of alcohol as a therapeutic agent. As a beverage, when constantly used, it is liable to cause obesity, gastric indigestion, arteriosclerosis, myocardial degeneration, chronic nephritis and cirrhosis of the liver. Its first action is undoubtedly as a food, if not too large amounts are taken, and therefore it is a protector of other food, especially of fat and starch. A habitue, then, especially if he has reached the age at which he normally adds weight, increases his tendency to obesity, and the first mistake in his nutrition is made. If lie takes too much alcohol when he eats or afterward, his digestion will be interfered with. Sooner or later, then, gastritis and stomach indigestion develop, with consequent intestinal indigestion. If lie takes strong alcohol, like whisky, oil an empty stomach, he may sooner or later cause serious disease of the mucous membrane of the stomach, first chronic gastritis, and later atrophy of the glands of the stomach.

Alcohol with meals which contain meat tends to the production of an increased amount of uric acid. Alcohol taken before meals on an empty stomach causes sudden vasodilatation after absorption. It goes quickly to the liver, irritates it, and little by little causes congestions of the liver, so that sooner or later sclerosis of this organ develops.

Alcohol probably causes arteriosclerosis not by its action per se, but indirectly by causing gastro-intestinal indigestion and insufficiency of the liver, as a result of which more toxins circulate in the blood, tending to produce arteriosclerosis. Sooner or later these irritants cause kidney irritation, and chronic interstitial nephritis may develop. just which process becomes the farthest advanced and finally kills the patient is an individual proposition and cannot be foretold. The finale may be cirrhosis of the liver, uremia, arteriosclerosis, apoplexy or myocarditis with dilatation or coronary disease.

While small, more or less undiluted closes of alcohol, as whisky or brandy, may cause quick stimulation of the heart by reflex irritation of the esophagus and stomach, vasodilatation occurs as soon as the alcohol is absorbed, and if large closes are absorbed, vasomotor paresis may occur, temporarily at least.

During acute fever processes with an increased pulse rate, provided shock or collapse is not present, small or medium-sized doses of alcohol, by dilating the peripheral blood vessels and increasing the peripheral circulation, may relieve the tension of the heart and slow the pulse by the equalization of the circulation. Some of this action may be due to the narcotic effect of alcohol on the cerebrum. Alcohol may thus in many instances act for good. Overdoses, as shown by cerebral excitation, flushing of the face and increased pulse rate, will do harm; in fact, many a patient with a serious illness, as typhoid fever or pneumonia, is made delirious by alcohol. Large doses of alcohol in shock or collapse are contraindicated.

Chronic overuse of alcohol may cause chronic myocarditis and fatty degeneration of the heart, with later weakening of the heart muscle and dilatation.

In acute alcohol poisoning the pulse may become very rapid and weak, and the patient may die of heart failure. This is often seen in delirium tremens. The administration in this condition of enormous doses of digitalis by the stomach is inexcusable, and the reason that such patients survive such digitalis poisoning is that the stomach does not absorb during this cardiac prostration.

A treatment as successful as any in this heart weakness in delirium tremens is morphin sulphate, 1/2 grain, and atropin, 1/15 grain, given hypodermically, with the administration of digitalis hypodermically for its later action on the heart. If the heart is contracting very rapidly, an ice-bag over the precordia will often quiet it. If the pulse is very weak, the cerebral sedatives more frequently used in delirium tremens, such as chloral, bromids, paraldehyd, etc., are generally contraindicated. A hot foot-bath and an ice-cap on the head sometimes aid in establishing a more general equalization of the circulation. It may often be necessary to administer strychnin, although if the patient is greatly excited it should be withheld as long as possible. For the same reason camphor, coffee and other cardiac stimulants which cause cerebral excitation should be withheld.

If the patient is in alcoholic coma, the pulse is generally slow, although it may be of low pressure unless the patient is otherwise diseased. Caffein or coffee is here indicated, and the patient should be kept warm lest he lose necessary heat. The stomach should be emptied by an emetic, often best by apomorphin hypodermically, unless the pulse is excessively weak. Strychnin may also be given, and digitalis, hypodermically, if it seems indicated. Camphor is another cardiac and cerebral stimulant that is valuable in these cases.

The treatment of an actual degeneration of the heart from overuse of alcohol is similar to the sane condition from other causes.

CAFFEIN

Caffein can irritate the heart and cause irregularity and tachycardia, especially in certain persons. In fact, some can never take a single cup of coffee without having an attack of palpitation, and many times when coffee and tea have been unsuspected by the patient as the cause of cardiac irritability, their removal from the diet has stopped the symptoms, and the heart has at once acted normally.

Caffein is a stimulant and tonic to the heart, increasing its rapidity and the strength of the contractions. It is also a cerebral stimulant, one of the most active that we possess among the drugs. It increases the blood pressure, principally by stimulating the vasomotor center and by increasing the heart strength. It acts as a diuretic, not only by increasing the circulatory force and blood pressure, but also by acting directly on the kidney. This action on the kidney contraindicates the use of caffein in any form, except in rare instances, when there is acute or chronic nephritis. The increased blood pressure caused by caffein also contraindicates its use when there is hypertension. Caffein first accelerates the heart and later may slow it and strengthen it; but if the dose is large or too frequently repeated, the apex of the heart ceases to relax properly and there is an interference with the contraction of the ventricles, the heart muscle becomes irritable, and a tachycardia may develop.

Therefore when a heart has serious lesions, whether of the myocardium or of the valves, with compensation only sufficient, the action of caffein in any form is contraindicated. The fact that it raises the blood pressure, thus increasing the force against which the heart must act, and that it irritates the heart muscle to more sturdy or irregular contraction, indicates that a patient with a heart lesion or with a nervously irritable heart should never drink tea and coffee or take caffein in any beverage.

Many patients cannot sleep for many hours after they have taken coffee or tea, as the cerebral stimulation of caffein is projected for hours after its ingestion. Caffein does not absorb so quickly and therefore does not act so quickly when taken in the form of tea and coffee as it does when taken as the drug or as a beverage which contains the alkaloid. Persons who are nervously irritable, excited and overstimulated cerebrally, with or without high blood pressure, should not take this cerebral and nervous excitant. This is true in early childhood and in youth, and continues true as age advances, in most persons. It is a crime to present caffein as a soda fountain beverage to children and young persons when the excitement of the age is such as already to overstimulate all nervous systems and all hearts.

A considerable majority of persons over 40 learn that they cannot drink tea or coffee with their evening meal without finding it difficult to sleep. Such patients, of course, should omit this stimulant.

Some patients have already recognized this fact and its cause; others must be told. The majority of adults are probably no worse and may be distinctly benefited by the morning cup of coffee and the noon coffee or tea, provided the amount taken is not large. It seems to be a fact that the drinking of coffee is on the increase, especially as to frequency. Certainly the five o'clock tea, with women, is on the increase, and we must deal with one more cerebral and nervous excitant in our consideration of what we shall do to slow this rapid age.

TOBACCO

In spite of the fact that a large number of men today do not smoke, more and more frequently every clinician has a patient who smokes too much. The accuracy with which he investigates these cases depends somewhat on his personal use of tobacco, and therefore his leniency toward a fellow user. Perhaps the percentage of young boys who smoke excessively is larger than the percentage of men. Whether or not the term "excessive" should be applied to any particular amount of tobacco consumed depends entirely on the person. What may be only a large amount for one person may be an excessive amount for another, and even one cigar a day may be too much for a person is as much for him as five or more cigars for another. If one is to judge by the internal revenue report it will appear that, in spite of the public school instruction as to the physiologic action of tobacco and its harm, and in spite of the antitobacco leagues, the consumption of tobacco is enormously on the increase.

Alexander Lambert [Footnote: Lambert, Alexander: Med. Rec., New York, Feb. 13, 1915] in studying periodic drinkers and alcoholics, finds that most patients are suffering from chronic tobacco poisoning, and if they stop their smoking, their drinking sometimes ceases automatically.

Howat [Footnote: Howat: Am. Jour. Physiol., February, 1916.] has shown that nicotin causes serious disturbances of the reflexes of the skin of frogs.

Edmunds and Smith [Footnote: Edmunds and Smith: Jour. Lab. and Clin. Med., February, 1916.] of Ann Arbor find that the livers of dogs have some power of destroying nicotin, but their studies did not show how tolerance to large doses of nicotin is acquired.

Neuhof [Footnote: Neuhof, Selian: Sino-Auricular Block Due to Tobacco Poisoning, Arch. Int. Med., May, 1916, p. 659.] describes a case of sino-auricular heart block due to tobacco poisoning. Intermittent claudication has been noted from the overuse of tobacco, as well as cramps in the muscles and of the legs.

A long series of investigations of the action of tobacco on high school boys and students of colleges seems to show that the age of graduation of smokers is older than that of nonsmokers, and that smokers require disciplinary measures more frequently than nonsmokers.

Some years ago investigation was made by Torrence, of the Illinois State Reformatory, in which there were 278 boys between the ages of 10 and 15 years. Ninety-two percent of these boys had the habit of smoking cigaretes, and 85 percent were classed as cigarete fiends.

The most important action of nicotin is on the circulation. Except during the stage when the person is becoming used to the tobacco habit, in which stage the heart is weakened and the vasomotor pressure lowered by his nausea and prostration, the blood pressure is almost always raised during the period of smoking.

The heart is frequently made more rapid and the blood pressure is certainly raised in an ordinary smoker, while even a novice may get at first an increase, but soon he may become depressed and have a lowering of the pressure. While a moderate smoker may have an increase of 10 mm. in blood pressure, an excessive smoker may show but little change. Perhaps this is because his heart muscle has become weakened. If the person's blood pressure is high, the heart may not increase in rapidity during smoking, and if he is nervous beforehand and is calmed by his tobacco, the pulse will be slowed. It has been shown that the blood pressure and pulse rate may be affected in persons sitting in a smoke-filled room, even though they themselves do not smoke. The length of time the increased pressure continues depends on the person, and it is this diminishing pressure that causes many to take another smoke. The heart is slowed by the action of nicotin on the vagi, as these nerves are stimulated both centrally and peripherally. An overdose of nicotin will paralyze the vagi. The heart action then becomes rapid and perhaps irregular. The heart muscle is first stimulated, and if too large a dose is taken, or too much in twenty-four hours, the muscle becomes depressed and perhaps debilitated. The consequence of such action on the heart muscle, sooner or later, is a dilation of the left ventricle if the overuse of the tobacco is continued.

There is, then, no possible opportunity for any discussion as to the action of tobacco on the circulation. Its action is positive, constantly occurs, and it is always to be considered. The only point at this issue is as to whether or not such an activity is of consequence to the individual. The active principle of tobacco is nicotin, besides which it contains an aromatic camphor-like substance, cellulose, resins, sugar, etc. Other products developed during combustion are carbon monoxid gas, a minute amount of prussic acid and in some varieties a considerable amount of furfurol, a poison. From any one cigar or cigaret but little nicotin is absorbed, else the user would be poisoned. It is generally considered that the best tobacco comes from Cuba, and in the United States from Virginia. While it has not been definitely shown that any stronger narcotic drug occurs in cigarets sold in this country, it still is of great interest to note that a user who becomes habituated to one particular brand will generally have no other, and the excessive cigaret-smoker will generally select the strongest brand of cigarets. The same is almost equally true of cigar smokers.

Besides the effect on the circulation, no one who uses tobacco can deny that it has a soothing, narcotic effect. If it did not have this quieting effect on the nervous system, the increased blood pressure would stimulate the cerebrum. Following a large meal, especially if alcohol has been taken, the blood vessels of the abdomen are more or less dilated by the digestion which is in process. During this period of lassitude it is possible that tobacco, through its contracting power, by raising the blood pressure in the cerebrum to the height at which the patient is accustomed, will stimulate him and cause him to be more able to do active mental work. On the other hand, if a person is nervously tired, irritable, or even muscularly weary, a cigar or several cigarets will increase his blood pressure, take away his circulatory tire, soothe his irritability, and stop temporarily his muscular pains or aches and muscle weariness. If the user of the tobacco has thorough control of his habit, is not working excessively, physically or mentally, has his normal sleep at night and therefore does not become weary from insomnia, he may use tobacco with sense and in the amount and frequency that is more or less harmless as far as he is concerned. If such a man, however, is sleepless, overworked or worried, if he has irregular meals or goes without his food, and has a series of "dinners," or drinks a good deal of alcohol, which gives him vasomotor relaxation, he finds a constantly growing need for a frequent smoke, and soon begins to use tobacco excessively. Or the young boy, stimulated by his associates, smokes cigarets more and more frequently until he uses them to excess.

Just what creates the intense desire for tobacco to the habitue has not been quite decided, but probably it is a combination of the irritation in the throat, especially in inhalers; of the desire for the rhythmic puffing which is a general cerebral and circulatory stimulant; for the increased vasomotor tension which many a patient feels the need of; for the narcotic, sedative, quieting effect on his brain or nerves; for the alluring comfort of watching the smoke curl into the air or for the quiet, contented sociability of smoking with associates. Probably all of these factors enter into the desire to continue the tobacco habit in those who smoke, so to speak, normally.

The abnormal smokers, or those who use tobacco excessively, have a more and more intense nervous desire or physical need of the narcotic or the circulatory stimulant effect of the tobacco, and, consequently, smoke more and more constantly. They are largely inhalers, and frequently cigaret fiends.

It is probable that tobacco smoked slowly and deliberately, when the patient is at rest, and when he is leading a lazy, inactive, nonhustling life, such as occurs in the warmer climates, is much less harmful than in our colder climates, where life is more active. Something at least seems to demonstrate that cigaret smoking is more harmful in our climate than in the tropics.

It has been shown by athletic records and by physicians' examinations of boys and young men in gymnasiums that perfect circulation, perfect respiration and perfect normal growth of the chest are not compatible with the use of tobacco during the growing period. It is also known that tobacco, except possibly in minute quantities, prevents the full athletic power, circulatorily and muscularly, of men who compete in any branch of athletics that requires prolonged effort.

The chronic inflammation of the pharynx and subacute or chronic irritation of the lingual tonsil, causing the tickling, irritating, dry cough of inhalers of tobacco, is too well known, to need description.

Many patients who oversmoke lose their appetites, have disturbances from inhibition of the gastric digestion, and may have an irregular action of the bowels from overstimulation of the intestines, since nicotin increases peristalsis. Such patients look sallow, grow thin and lose weight. These are the kind of patients who smoke while they are dressing in the morning, on the way to their meals, to and from their business, and not only before going to bed, but also after they are in bed. It might be a question as to whether such patients do not need conservators. The use of tobacco in that way is absolutely inexcusable, if the patient is not mentally warped. Cancer of the mouth caused by smoking, blindness from the overuse of tobacco, muscular trembling, tremors, muscle cramps and profuse perspiration of the hands and feet are all recognized as being caused by tobacco poisoning, but such symptoms need not be further described here.

The reason for which physicians most frequently must stop their patients from using tobacco, however, is that the heart itself has become affected by the nicotin action. The heart muscle is never strengthened by nicotin, but is always weakened by excessive indulgence in nicotin, the nerves of the heart being probably disturbed, if not actually injured. The positive symptoms of the overuse of tobacco on the heart are attacks of palpitation on exertion lasting perhaps but a short time, sharp, stinging pains in the region of the heart, less firmness of the apex beat, perhaps irregularity of the heart, and cold hands and feet. Clammy perspiration frequently occurs, more especially on the hands. Before the heart muscle actually weakens, the blood pressure has been increased more or less constantly, perhaps permanently, until such time as the left ventricle fails. The left ventricle from tobacco alone, without any other assignable cause, may become dilated and the mitral valve become insufficient. Before the heart has been injured to this extent the patient learns that he cannot lie on his left side at night without discomfort, that exertion causes palpitation, and that he frequently has an irregularly acting heart and an irregular pulse. He may have cramps in his legs, leg-aches and cold hands and feet from an imperfect systemic circulation. In this condition if tobacco is entirely stopped, and the patient put on digitalis and given the usual careful advice as to eating, drinking, exertion, exercise and rest, such a heart will generally improve, acquire its normal tone, and the mitral valve become again sufficient, and to all intents and purposes the patient becomes well.

On the other hand, a heart under the overuse of tobacco may show no signs of disability, but its reserve energy is impaired and when a serious illness occurs, when an operation with the necessary anesthesia must be endured or when any other sudden strain is put on this heart, it goes to pieces and fails more readily than a heart that has not been so damaged.

If a patient does not show such cardiac weakness but has high tension, the danger of hypertension is increased by his use of tobacco, and certainly in hypertension tobacco should be prohibited. The nicotin is doing two things for him that are serious: first, it is raising his blood pressure, and second, it will sooner or later weaken his heart, which may be weakened by the high blood pressure alone. Nevertheless a patient who is a habitual user of tobacco and has circulatory failure noted more especially about or during convalescence from a serious illness, particularly pneumonia, may best be improved by being allowed to smoke at regular intervals and in the amount that seems sufficient. Such patients sometimes rapidly improve when their previous circulatory weakness has been a subject of serious worry. Even such patients who were actually collapsed have been saved by the use of tobacco.

Whether the tobacco in a given patient shall be withdrawn absolutely, or only modified in amount, depends entirely on the individual case. As stated above, no rule can be laid down as to what is enough and what is too much. Theoretically, two or three cigars a day is moderate, and anything more than five cigars a day is excessive; even one cigar a day may be too much.

MISCELLANEOUS DISTURBANCES

SIMPLE HYPERTROPHY

Like any other muscular tissue, the heart hypertrophies when it has more work to do, provided this work is gradually increased and the heart is not strained by sudden exertion. To hypertrophy properly the heart must go into training. This training is necessary in valvular lesions after acute endocarditis or myocarditis, and is the reason that the return to work must be so carefully graduated. When the heart is hypertrophied sufficiently and compensation is perfect, a reserve power must be developed by such exercise as represented by the Nauheim, Oertel or Schott methods. Anything that increases the peripheral resistance causes the left ventricle to hypertrophy. Anything that increases the resistance in the lungs causes the right ventricle to hypertrophy. The right ventricle hypertrophy caused by mitral lesions has already been sufficiently discussed. The right ventricle also hypertrophies in emphysema, after repeated or prolonged asthma attacks, perhaps generally in neglected pleurisies with effusion, in certain kinds of tuberculosis, and whenever there is increased resistance in the lung tissue or in the chest cavity.

The term "simple hypertrophy" is generally restricted to hypertrophy of the left ventricle without any cardiac excuse—the hypertrophy by hypertension and hard physical labor. It is well recognized that it hypertrophies with hypertension and with chronic interstitial nephritis. It also becomes hypertrophied when the subject drinks largely of liquid—water or beer—and overloads his blood vessels and increases the work the heart must do. This kind of hypertrophy develops slowly because the resistance in the circulation is gradual or intermittent. In athletes and in soldiers who are required to march long distances, hypertrophy generally occurs. This hypertrophy, if slowly developed by gradual, careful training, is normal and compensatory. In effort too long sustained, especially in those untrained in that kind of effort, and even in the trained if the effort is too long continued, the left ventricle will become dilated and the usual symptoms of that condition occur. Such dilatation is always more or less serious. It may be completely recovered from, and it may not be. Therefore it proper understanding of the physics of the circulation by the medical trainer of young men to decide whether or not one should compete in a prolonged effort, as a rowing race, for instance, is essential. It is wrong for any young athlete to have an incurable condition occur from competition.

Sometimes simple hypertrophy of the left ventricle occurs from various kinds of conditions that increase the peripheral circulation. It may occur from oversmoking, from the mertisc of coffee aid tea, from certain kinds of physical labor, or from high tension mental work. It is a part of the story of hypertension. Many times such patients, as well as occasionally trained athletes, and sometimes patients with arteriosclerosis or chronic interstitial nephritis complain of unpleasant throbbing sensations of the heart added to these sensations are a feeling of fulness in the head, flushing of the face, and possibly dizziness—all symptoms not only of hypertension but of too great cardiac activity. Various drugs used to stimulate the heart may cause this condition; when digitalis is given and is not indicated or is given in overdosage, these symptoms occur.

The treatment is simply to lower the diet, cause catharsis, give hot baths, stop the tobacco, tea and coffee, stop the drinking of large amounts of liquid at any one time, and administer bromids and perhaps nitroglycerin, when all the symptoms of simple hypertrophy will, temporarily at least, disappear.

If the heart is enlarged from hypertrophy, if it is the right ventricle that is the most hypertrophied, the apex is not only pushed to the left, but the beat may be rather diffuse, as the enlarged right ventricle will prevent the apex from acting close to the surface of the chest. If the left ventricle is the most hypertrophied, the apex is also to the left, but the impact is very decided and the aortic closure is accentuated.

SIMPLE DILATATION

The term "simple dilatation" may be applied to the dilatation of one or both ventricles when there is no valvular lesion and when the condition may not be called broken compensation. The compensation has been sufficiently discussed. Dilatation of the heart occurs when there is increased resistance to the outflow of the blood front the ventricle, or when the ventricle is overfilled with blood and the muscular wall is unable to compete with the increased work thrown on it. In other words, it may be weakened by myocarditis or fatty degeneration; or it may be a normal heart that has sustained a strain; or it may be a hypertrophied heart that has become weakened. Heart strain is of frequent occurrence. It occurs in young men from severe athletic effort; it occurs in older persons from some severe muscle strain, and it may even occur from so simple an effort as rapid walking by one who is otherwise diseased and whose heart is unable to sustain even this extra work. All of the conditions which have been enumerated as causing simple hypertrophy may have dilatation as a sequence.

Degeneration and disturbance of the heart muscle and cardiac dilatation are found more and more frequently at an earlier age than such conditions should normally occur. Several factors are at work in causing this condition. In the first place, infants and children are now being saved though they may have inherited, or acquired, a diminished withstanding power against disease and against the strain and vicissitudes of adult life. Other very important factors in causing the varied fortes of cardiac disturbances are the rapidity and strenuousness of a business and social life, and competitive athletics in school and college, to say nothing of the oversmoking and excessive dancing of many.

The symptoms of heart strain, if the condition is acute, are those of complete prostration, lowered blood pressure, and a sluggishly, insufficiently acting heart. The heart is found enlarged, the apex beat diffuse and there may be a systolic blow at the mitral or tricuspid valve. Sometimes, although the patient recognizes that he has hurt himself and strained his heart, he is not prostrated, and the full symptoms do not occur for several hours or perhaps several days, although the patient realizes that he is progressively growing weaker and more breathless.

The treatment of this acute or gradual dilatation is absolute rest, with small doses of digitalis gradually but slowly increased, and when the proper dosage is decided on, administered at that dosage but once a day. Cardiac stimulants should not be given, except when faintness or syncope has occurred, and if strychnin is used, it should be in small closes. The heart nay completely recover its usual powers, but subsequently it is more readily strained again by any thoughtless laborious effort. The patient must be warned as carefully as though he had a valvular lesion and had recovered from a broken compensation, and his life should be regulated accordingly, at least for some months. If he is young, and the heart completely and absolutely recovers, the force of the circulation may remain as strong as ever.

Sometimes the heart strain is not so severe, and after a few hours of rest and quiet the patient regains complete cardiac power and is apparently as well as ever; but for some time subsequently his heart more easily suffers strain.

Chronic dilatation of the heart, However, perhaps not sufficient to cause edema, slowly and insidiously develops from persistent strenuosity, or from the insidious irritations caused by absorbed toxins due to intestinal indigestion. A fibrosis of the heart muscle and of the arterioles gradually develops, and the heart muscle sooner or later feels the strain.

It is now very frequent for the physician, in his office, to hear the patient say, "Doctor, I am not sick, but just tired," or, "I get tired on the least exertion." We do not carefully enough note the condition of the heart in our patients who are just "weary," or even when they show beginning cardiovascular-renal trouble.

The primary symptoms of this condition of myocardial weakening are slight dyspnea on least exertion; slight heart pain; slight edema above the ankles; often some increased heart rapidity, sometimes without exertion; after exertion the heart does not immediately return to its normal frequency; slight dyspnea on least exertion after eating; flushing of the face or paleness around the mouth, and more or less dilatation of the veins of the hands. All of these are danger signals which may not be especially noted at first by the individual; but, if he presents himself to his physician, such a story should cause the latter not only to make a thorough physical examination, but also to note particularly the size of the heart.

It a roentgenographic and fluoroscopic examination cannot be made, careful percussion, noting the region of the apex beat, noting the rapidity and action of the heart on sitting, standing and lying, and noting the length of time it takes while resting, after exertion, for the speed of the heart to slacken, will show the heart strength.

Slight dilatation being diagnosed, the treatment is as follows

1. Rest, absolute if needed, and the prohibition of all physical exercise and of all business cares.

2. Reduction in the amount of food, which should be of the simplest. Alcohol should be stopped, and the amount of tea, coffee and tobacco reduced.

3. If medication is needed, strychnin sulphate, 1/40, or 1/30 grain three times a day, acid the tincture of digitalis in from 5 to 10 drop doses twice a day will aid the heart to recover its tone.

Such treatment, when soon applied to a slowly dilating and weakening heart, will establish at least a temporary cure and will greatly- prolong life.

If these hearts are not diagnosed and properly treated, such patients are liable to die suddenly of "heart failure," of acute stomach dilatation, or of angina pectoris. Furthermore, unsuspected dilated hearts are often the cause of sudden deaths during the first forty-eight hours of pneumonia.

Small doses of digitalis are sufficient in these early cases. If more heart pain is caused, the dose of digitalis is too large, or it is contraindicated. Digitalis need not be long given in this condition, especially as Cohen, Fraser and Jamison [Footnote: Cohen, Fraser and Jamison: Jour. Exper. Med., June, 1915.] have shown by the electrocardiograph that its effect on the heart may last twenty- two days, and never lasts a shorter time than five days. They also found that when digitalis is given by the mouth, the electrocardiograph showed that its full activity was not reached until from thirty-six to forty-eight hours after it had been taken. From these scientific findings it will he seen that if it is necessary to give a second course of treatment with digitalis, within two weeks at least from the time the last close of digitalis was given, the dose of this drug should be much smaller than when it was first administered.

Owing to our strenuous life, if persons over 40 would present themselves for a heart and other physical examination once or twice a year there would not be so many sudden deaths of those thought to be in good health. It may be a fact as asserted by many of our best but depressing and pessimistic clinicians, that chronic myocarditis and fatty degeneration of the heart cannot be diagnosed by any special set of symptoms or signs. However, it is a fact that a tolerably accurate estimate of the heart strength can be made by a careful physician, and if danger signals are noted and signs of probable heart weakness are present, life may be long saved by good treatment or management rigorously carried out. The patient must cooperate, and to get him to do this he must be tactfully warned of his condition. Many, such patients, noting their impaired ability, do not seek medical advice, but think all they need is more exercise; hence they walk, golf, and dance to excess and to their cardiac undoing.

HEART IN ACUTE DISEASE

ACUTE DILATATION OF THE HEART IN ACUTE DISEASE

It has for a long time been recognized that in all acute prolonged illness the heart fails, sooner or later, often without its having been attacked by the disease. The prolonged high temperature causes the heart to beat more rapidly, while the toxins produced by the fever process cause muscle degeneration of the heart or a myocarditis, and at the same time the nutrition of the heart becomes impaired either by improper feeding or by the imperfect metabolism of the food given; hence the heart muscle becomes weakened, and cardiac failure or cardiac relaxation or dilatation occurs.

The specific germ of the disease, or the toxin elaborated by this germ, may be especially depressant to the heart, as in diphtheria, or the germ may be particularly prone to locate in the heart, as in rheumatism and pneumonia. But all feverish processes, sooner or later, if sufficiently prolonged, cause serious cardiac weakness and more or less dilatation.

Just exactly what changes take place in the muscle fibers of the heart in some of these fevers has not been decided. Whether an albuminous or parenchymatous degeneration of the muscle fibers or a fatty degeneration occurs, whether there is a real myocarditis that always precedes the dilatation, or whether the weakening and loss of muscle fibers or a diminished power of the muscle fibers occurs without inflammation, dilatation of the heart is always a factor to be considered, and frequently occurs in acute disease.

While it is denied that acute dilatation can occur in a sound heart, at the latter end of a serious illness the heart is never sound, and acute dilatation can most readily occur, though fortunately it is generally preventable. When the dilatation occurs suddenly, as indicated by a fluttering heart, a low tension, rapid pulse, dyspnea and perhaps cyanosis with venous stasis in the capillaries, death is imminent, although such patients may be saved by proper aid. Even when the dilatation is slower, as evidenced by a gradually increasing rapidity of the heart and a gradually lowering blood pressure, and with more evidences of exhaustion, death may occur from such heart failure in spite of all treatment.

Unless a patient dies from accident, as from a hemorrhage, from cerebral pressure or from some organic lesion in acute disease, the physician frequently feels that if he can hold the power and force of the circulation for several hours or days, the patient will recover from the disease, for in most acute diseases the patient has a good chance of recovery if his circulation will only hold out until the crisis has occurred or until the disease is ready to end by lysis. Therefore anything during the disease that tends to sustain, nourish, quiet and guard the heart means so much more chance of recovery, whatever else may or may not be done for the disease itself.

The best treatment of dilatation of the heart in acute disease is its prevention, and to prevent it means to recognize the condition which can cause it. These are

1. Prolonged high temperature. A short-lived temperature, even if high, is not serious. Prolonged temperature of even 103 F. or more is serious, and even that of 101 is serious if too long continued.

2. Exertion and excitement. Every possible means should be inaugurated to prevent muscular exertion and strain of the patient while in bed. Proper help in lifting and turning the patient should be employed, the bed-pan should be used, proper feeding methods should be adopted, and friends should be excluded so that the patient may not be excited by conversation.

3. Bad feeding. The diet should of course be sufficient, for the patient and proper for the disease, but any diet which causes a large amount of gas in the stomach, or tympanites, is harmful to the patient's circulation, to say nothing of any other harm, such as indigestion may do. All of the nutriments needed to keep the body in perfect condition should be given to a patient who is ill; in some manner he should receive the proper amounts of iron, salt, calcium, starch, protein, sugar and water.

4. Intestinal sluggishness. This means not only that tympanites should not be allowed, but also that necessary laxatives should be given. It would be wrong to prostrate a patient with frequent saline purgatives, but the bowels must move at least once every other day, generally better daily; and if the case is one of typhoid fever, they should be moved by some carefully selected laxative, and after the bowels have sufficiently moved, the diarrhea should be stopped by 1/10 grain of morphin, and the next day the bowels properly moved again.

5. Depressant drugs. In this age of cardiac failure, heart depressants of all types, and especially the synthetic products, should be given only with careful judgment, and, never frequently repeated or long continued.

6. Pain. This is one of the most serious depressants a heart has to combat; acute pain must not be allowed, and prolonged subacute pain must be stopped. Even peripheral troublesome irritations must be removed, as tending to wear out a heart which has all of the trouble it can endure.

7. Insomnia. Nothing rests a heart or recuperates a heart more than sleep. Insomnia and acute disease make a combination which will wear a heart out more quickly than any other combination. Sleep, then, must be produced in the best, easiest and safest manner possible.

8. A too speedy return to activity. The convalescence must be prolonged until the heart is able to sustain the work required of it.

The treatment of gradual dilatation in acute disease has been sufficiently discussed under the subject of acute myocarditis. The treatment of acute dilatation is practically the same as the treatment of shock plus whatever treatment must coincidently be given to a patient for the disease with which he is suffering. The treatment of shock will be discussed under a separate heading.

THE HEART IN PNEUMONIA

As pneumonia heads the list of the causes of death in this country, and as the heart fails so quickly, sometimes almost in the beginning in pneumonia, a special discussion of the management of the heart in this disease is justifiable.

Acute lobar pneumonia may kill a patient in twenty-four or forty-eight hours; lie may live for a week and die of heart failure or toxemia, or he may live for several weeks and die of cardiac weakness. If he has double pneumonia be may die almost of suffocation. It is today just as frequent to see a slowly developing and slowly resolving pneumonia as to see one of the sthenic type that attacks one lobe with a rush, has a crisis in a seven, eight or nine days, and then a rapid resolution. In fact the asthenic type, in which different parts of the lung are involved but not necessarily confined to or even equivalent to one lobe, is perhaps the most frequent form of pneumonia.

The serious acute congestion of the lung in sthenic pneumonia in a full-blooded, sturdy person with high tension pulse may be relieved by cardiac sedatives, vasodilators, brisk purging, or by the relaxing effect of antipyretics. Venesection is often the best treatment.

When the sputum almost from the first is tinged with venous blood, or even when the sputum is very bloody, of the prune-juice variety, the heart is in serious trouble, and the right ventricle has generally become weak and possibly dilated. The heart may have been diseased and therefore is unable to overcome the pressure in the lungs during the congestion and consolidation.

There is a great difference in the belief of clinicians as to the best treatment for this condition. It would seem to be a positive indication for digitalis, and good-sized doses of digitalis given correctly, provided always that the preparation of the drug used is active, are good and, many times, efficient treatment. Small doses of strychnin may be of advantage, and camphor may be of value. In the condition described, however, reliance should be placed on digitalis. Later in the disease when the heart begins to fail, perhaps the cause is a myocarditis. In this condition digitalis would not work so well and might do harm. It is quite possible that the difference between digitalis success and digitalis nonsuccess or harm may be as to whether or not a myocarditis is present.

If the expectoration is not of the prune-juice variety and is not more than normally bloody, or in other words, typically pneumonic, and the heart begins to fail, especially if there is no great amount of consolidation, the left ventricle is in trouble as much as the right, if not more. In this case all of the means described above for the prevention of any dilatation of the heart will be means of preventing dilatation from the pneumonia, if possible. The treatment advisable for this gradually failing heart is camphor; strychnin in not too large doses, at the most 1/10 grain hypodermically once in six hours; often ergot intramuscularly once in six hours for two or three doses and then once in twelve hours; plenty of fresh air, or perhaps the inhalation of oxygen. Oxygen does not cure pneumonia, but may relieve a dyspnea and aid a heart until other drugs have time to act.

If there is insomnia, morphin in small doses will not only cause sleep, but also not hurt the heart. In the morning hours of the day the value of caffein as a cardiac stimulant and vasocontractor, either in the form of caffein or as black coffee, should be remembered. Strophanthin may be given intravenously.

One of the greatest cares in the treatment of heart failure in pneumonia should be not to give too many drugs or to do too much.

SHOCK

The treatment of shock will probably always be unsatisfactory as the cause is so varied, and, although circulatory prostration and vasomotor paresis always constitute the acute condition, the physiologic health of the heart and blood vessels is so varied. The patient in shock has low temperature, low blood pressure, and a pulse either rapid or slow, but excessively feeble; the face is pale, the surface of the body cold, and there is more or less clammy perspiration; there may be dyspnea and cardiac anxiety, or the patient may hardly breathe.

An acute cause, as terrible pain or hemorrhage, must of course be stopped immediately. There is more or less anemia of the brain, and therefore the legs and perhaps the lower part of the body should be elevated. It may even be wise to drive the blood from the legs by Esmarch bandages into the rest of the circulation. As there is always more or less paresis and dilatation of the large veins of the splanchnic system, a tight bandage about the abdomen is of great advantage in raising the blood pressure to the safety mark.

Strophanthin, given intravenously, is valuable as a quick restorative of the heart. Digitalis is so slow that it is of little value in an emergency. Camphor hypodermically, and hot liquids (nothing is better than black coffee) given by the mouth, are valuable remedies. The camphor may be repeated frequently. Strychnin, the long-used stimulant, should generally be given, but in not too large doses and not too frequently repeated; 1/30 grain hypodermically is generally a large enough dose; this dose may be repeated in three or four hours, but should ordinarily not be given oftener than once in six hours. An aseptic preparation of ergot given intramuscularly is most efficient in raising the blood pressure and aiding the heart. One dose of brandy or whisky may do no harm. Alcohol, however, should not be pushed.

A most important procedure in all kinds of shock is to surround the patient with dry heat, hot-water bags, and hot flannels; gentle friction of the arms and legs, unless the patient is too exhausted, may be of benefit. A hot-water bag to the heart is always a stimulant. Sometimes friction over the base of the heart in the region of the auricles is of benefit.

If the collapse is not acute and there is gradual profound prostration, or if the patient is improved but still in a serious condition of shock, too energetic measures must not be used; neither should too many drugs be administered, or drugs in too large doses. Absolute quiet and the administration of liquid nourishment in but small amounts at a time are essential.

The hypodermic administration of epinephrin solutions, 1:10,000, or solutions of pituitary extract, 1:10,000, should be considered; they are often valuable.

If the shock occurs in ether or chloroform anesthesia, the vasopressor stimulating effect of inhalations of carbon dioxid gas may be considered, as advised by Henderson."

If the shock is due to hemorrhage and the hemorrhage has ceased, a transfusion of physiologic saline solution is generally indicated. Transfusion of blood under the same conditions is still better. Rarely is transfusion indicated in shock from other causes; it often adds to the difficulty rather than improves it. Occasionally if shock is decided to be due to a toxemia, the toxin may be diluted by the withdrawal of a small amount of blood and the transfusion of an equal amount of saline solution.

ACUTE DILATATION OF THE STOMACH

This condition is not well understood, nor is its frequence known, but not a few instances of shock are due to dilatation of this organ. The shock to the heart may be a reflex one through the pneumogastric nerves.

It perhaps not infrequently occurs after abdominal operations and is more or less serious, the symptoms being persistent vomiting, upper abdominal distention and collapse. The vomiting is of bloody or coffee-ground material.

Sometimes the ordinary treatment of the collapse and washing out the stomach save the patient; at other times the patient with this series of symptoms dies in spite of all treatment.

It has been shown that acute dilatation of the stomach may occur in pneumonia, and may be one of the causes of cardiac collapse in pneumonia.

When the condition is diagnosed, the treatment would be that of shock plus abdominal bandage and washing out the stomach with warm solutions, if the patient is not too collapsed, or at any rate the frequent administration of hot water in small quantities.

Sometimes when the stomach is dilated the pylorus becomes insufficient, and bile regurgitates into the stomach, and is a cause of the profound nausea and vomiting arid the subsequent collapse. In these cases

114. Henderson: Am. Jour. Physiol., February and April, 1909. not infrequently small doses of dilute hydrochloric acid seem to aid the pylorus to maintain its normal contraction, the regurgitation of bile does not take place, and the stomach may soon acquire a more normal muscle tone. Not infrequently when a stomach is in this kind of trouble and all the foods are rejected, and yet the patient seriously needs nourishment, a warm, thin cereal, as oatmeal or gruel or something similar, may be retained. Such patients, as has been repeatedly stated, need starch as soon as possible, lest an acidosis develop.

In these vomiting and collapse cases the hypodermic administration of morphin and atropin will not only stop the vomiting, at least temporarily, but will also give necessary rest. The dose of morphin need not be large, and the atropin may prevent nausea from the drug.

ANESTHESIA IN HEART DISEASE

While no physician likes to give an anesthetic to a patient who has valvular disease of the heart, and no surgeon cares to operate on such a patient unless operation is absolutely necessary, still in valvular disease with good compensation the prognosis of either ether or chloroform narcosis is good.

When there are evidences of chronic myocarditis or a history of broken compensation and the borderline of compensation and dilatation is very narrow, or when there is arteriosclerosis, the danger from an anesthetic and an operation is much greater; it may be serious, in fact, and the decision must be made whether or not the operation is absolutely necessary. Under any circumstances it is understood that the anesthetist must be an expert, as there can be no carelessness and nothing but the best of judgment in causing anesthesia when there is cardiac defect.

The anesthetic to select is a subject for careful decision, as one cannot assert which anesthetic is the best.

While chloroform seems occasionally to cause a fatty degeneration of the heart, or if given too rapidly at first may cause sudden death, especially in cardiac weakness, ether has its disadvantages, owing to the increased tension (especially if there is likely to be much valvular or cerebral excitement), and the greater amount of ether that must be given, with the attendant danger to the kidneys, which may have been disturbed from the cardiac conditions. Generally, however, the better method is perhaps to administer first chloroform to the point of producing sleep and then to change to ether, the first mild chloroform narcosis preventing the ether from causing acute stimulation, and ether being better for the operation, as it is more of a stimulant. Some anesthetists believe that it is better to administer morphin, with perhaps atropin hypodermically before the anesthesia, and then to use ether. Nitrous oxid gas would be contraindicated as tending to increase arterial pressure, and therefore endanger a damaged heart; it is a serious danger to damaged blood vessels.